DETACHED LOVE

TRANSFORMING YOUR HEART SO THAT
YOU CAN TRANSFORM YOUR MIND

CORDELIA A. GAFFAR

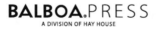

BALBOA.PRESS
A DIVISION OF HAY HOUSE

Balboa Press books may be ordered through booksellers or by contacting:

Balboa Press
A Division of Hay House
1663 Liberty Drive
Bloomington, IN 47403
www.balboapress.com
844-682-1282

Because of the dynamic nature of the Internet, any web addresses or links contained in this book may have changed since publication and may no longer be valid. The views expressed in this work are solely those of the author and do not necessarily reflect the views of the publisher, and the publisher hereby disclaims any responsibility for them.

The author of this book does not dispense medical advice or prescribe the use of any technique as a form of treatment for physical, emotional, or medical problems without the advice of a physician, either directly or indirectly. The intent of the author is only to offer information of a general nature to help you in your quest for emotional and spiritual well-being. In the event you use any of the information in this book for yourself, which is your constitutional right, the author and the publisher assume no responsibility for your actions.

Any people depicted in stock imagery provided by Getty Images are models, and such images are being used for illustrative purposes only.
Certain stock imagery © Getty Images.

Print information available on the last page.

ISBN: 978-1-9822-5786-6 (sc)
ISBN: 978-1-9822-5787-3 (e)

Library of Congress Control Number: 2020921628

Balboa Press rev. date: 11/09/2020

CONTENTS

ACKNOWLEDGEMENTS

First and foremost, I share this book with the world in the name of Allah, the Most Compassionate, the Most Merciful. I dedicate this book to my six children because parenting and loving you has encouraged me to do my research and the work to show up powerfully for you and myself. I love you with all of my heart and soul. I also want to acknowledge my community, readers, clients and followers who I seek to serve at the highest level. I appreciate and acknowledge Devon Pollard, Carleeka Basnight-Menendez and Kisa Davis for giving me permission to share your stories. Additionally, I appreciate reviews by Rhonda Farah, Anita Hawkins and Robin Rose Benett.

I am extending my deepest gratitude to Devon Bandison for generously and beautifully writing the foreword.

FOREWORD

If you could be anybody who would you be?

I remember contemplating this question throughout my childhood and early adulthood. It started becoming a guiding question for me as a child, "who do you want to be?" I remember dreaming of one day becoming a professional and collegiate athlete; and after receiving a basketball scholarship I was able to live out part of that dream. After school, I then became focused on finding what success in the "real world" looked like. Shortly after getting into the "rat race" of the working world, I was given a gift like no other time in my life.

It was fatherhood.

Up until that point in my life there was nothing that impacted my life and so fundamentally touched every inch of my soul like the profound love and responsibility that came with being a father.

The question of "If I could be anybody who would I be?" looked very different to me all of a sudden. Until then the answer rested in some form of outward success (great basketball career, great corporate career, money, etc) mostly defined by people who had come before me. Well-meaning mentors, and friends had often shared with me some version of what success looked like to them. I hadn't really taken the time to slow down the question for myself.

Fatherhood did that for me. For the first time in my life, there was something that I was in touch with that reached far beyond anything that "success" in the material world could ever give me. I knew I was connected to something bigger than me, something that had always been with me throughout my life. I just never slowed down enough to acknowledge or nurture it. It was an inner knowing, a commitment to transforming who I BE. It was the release of years of conditioning. In many ways the birth of our daughter was a rebirth for me.

At that moment, I looked at the question with a different lens and it no longer looked the same. I had realized that the searching outside of myself for "who I would be" was no longer a worthy search. The more meaningful inquiry was the searching within for who I already was all along.

If I stripped away all the conditioning and unlearned all that was left unquestioned, "who would I discover?" When I slowed down to the speed of life and listened to that subtle whisper, that guide who has been with me all my life, what would I see as possible? One of my favorite quotes is from Mozart and my best New York paraphrase of the quote is that "music isn't in the notes, music is in the space between the notes." If music was just note after note it would be noise. How many of us live our lives with all the noise continually playing- in our heads? The noise that plays in the stories we tell about ourselves and others. The noise that turns what's possible into appearing impossible.

Over the early years, before self exploration I'd lived with a lot of noise in between my ears that told me things like:

> "you're not enough!"
> "who are you to do that?
> "you can't say that because they'll think you're cocky"
> "who do you think you are?"

That noise often prevents us from stepping into our divine, our greatness, the realm of creating the possible from the IMpossible.

Where has that noise held you back in your life? In your relationships? In your career?

Has that noise screamed "play small" at times when you knew inside that you had so much more to give? I know it did for me, until it didn't. Now and again, that noise tries to creep in and it no longer holds me back.

When I finally learned how to slow down and allow myself to listen to the "space between the notes." my life transformed. Possibility was everywhere, scarcity was nowhere- life, love and abundance was limitless.

Over the next 20 years I've dedicated my life to helping people answer a new question. The question is simple-

If you really knew how amazingly powerful you truly are, who would you be and what would you do with this wonderful life of yours?

I've spent countless hours studying and learning from some of the greatest teachers and gurus in the world of personal transformation and human potential. This work has taken me all across the globe serving people of all walks of life. I've been fortunate enough to ask this powerful question through a TED talk, a best selling book as well as a global community of people who are making an impact in the world.

And while Fatherhood is still front and center, at the core of all who I BE- I am grateful to be a part of personal transformation for women, men, families and leaders around the world.

Throughout all of this work, one of the things I love the most is coming across people who are truly inspiring. Inspiring in the latin root of the word *Spiro which means to breathe life into.* People who breathe life into the rooms they enter and the spaces they share with others. Through words, actions, and a way of Being.

Which is how I can best describe my not so chance encounter in meeting Cordelia Gaffar. I was hosting an online event called Co-Creating The Bridge, which brought people together from all over the world. The conversation looked at race with the mission to transform what it means to be human. It was big work and a big conversation that led to discussions that were often passionate and energized. And then a woman came onto the video call- cutting through all the noise, emotions, and exchanges. And when it was her time to talk, she paused and simply said "let's all take a moment and just breathe." It was such a powerful moment- picture 100's of people collectively pausing and breathing in what seemed like perfect synchronicity. It was oneness, a connectedness of the human spirit that seemed so perfectly aligned. I was in AWE of the moment and intrigued by the woman who helped create that moment.

What happened was a glimpse into the power of the "space between the notes" that Mozart was talking about. That woman who appeared and created this profound moment in time was Cordelia Gaffar. In that one moment the entire energy and love in that room expanded. It was magical, and I saw this powerful woman operate in that divine space between the notes. In that space she breathed life into that room.

From that moment on, I knew that I would become friends with Cordelia and learn more about her profoundly deep work. When she told me she was writing a book I wanted to get my hands on it and start reading it immediately. That book which you now hold in your hands takes the magic that the people in that room felt that night and brings it to life.

Right now, at this moment you are holding more than another book, you have a system that gives you access to self expression and freedom in your life. If I had this book 25 years ago, it would have saved me years of study because **Detached Love: Transforming Your Heart So That You Can Transform Your Mind** is a story about all of us. It takes the reader on a journey of love, laughter, heartbreak, compassion in a way that allows us to look within for our own answers.

Cordelia so eloquently takes her own life learnings and from it created a system that can help you transform your own life. The words will come to life and allow you to quit the noise and listen in the space between the notes. **Detached Love: Transforming Your Heart So That You Can Transform Your Mind** is a story about breaking down what no longer serves us in our lives, in order to live and be our best in all that we do. The system that is shared throughout the book gives you a pathway to breakthroughs in any areas that have been holding you back in your life, relationships and career.

What I love about this book is that Cordelia puts her own heart on the line, giving you a look into what it means to be truly vulnerable and authentic. You will find yourself questioning your own limiting beliefs and be left with an access to freedom and self expression like you've never experienced. By opening up the curtain into her journey, her system of self nurturing and her Replenish Me ™process, Cordelia so generously points you in a direction and leaves the path in which you take up to you.

In each chapter, you will receive practical applications that will empower you to release anything holding you back, restructure, refresh and replenish in a way that gives you access to your power and rebirth by breathing life into all that you do.

Now I ask you the question:

If you really knew how amazingly powerful you truly are, who would you be and what would you do with this wonderful life of yours?

The pages you are about to read, will bring out the clarity and commitment that will be required to live it out in your answer.

Put your seatbelt on, strap in and welcome to one of the most inspiring journeys of your life!

Devon Bandison, MPA

www.devonbandison.com

The Game Changer Coach

Author, *"Fatherhood is Leadership"*

INTRODUCTION

Geography of Emotions

As the realization of another poor choice hit my body I began to feel nauseous. I tried to stifle my tears but they were relentless and began to fall anyway. With every hot drop, my skin sizzled, and my body shook. As I tried to prevent dry heaving a full abdominal cramp seized my core, trickled up my shoulders and wreaked havoc on my nerves which then went full attack on my hips. I experienced a combination of menstrual cramps, fever, and the flu as tears gushed from my eyes and my mind processed the realization that I had identified yet another person to release from my life.

If we pay attention, our bodies tell us there is something wrong. It could be the words of a conversation that trigger the physical responses I have described or a thought. In this case, it was a conversation with a person I considered a friend. I was in absolute shock that someone could be so indifferent, condescending, and oblivious at the same time.

What I experienced shows how the geography of the energy centers work. Our energy centers can express emotions and ailments simultaneously and each occupies a special place in our bodies. The energy center for anger is our stomach, and the one for carrying other people's stuff is in our shoulders. The energy center for resentment is in our joints and for a lack of support in the hips. My grief and feeling of betrayal hit me first in my heart, causing the tears, shaking, and dry heaving. I hit all the stops on the map of the geography of our emotions at the same time after one brief interaction.

Before I had any thought to confront, or could lash out, or discuss the situation with the other party, I became overwhelmingly aware of my body symptoms so I combined self-love with a variety of other methods to heal my emotions. I took a walk but because the extreme emotions of confusion and anger were intertwined I also released using outer manipulation or massage and reflexology with my toes. Unconsciously, I headed for nutritious food and hydration. I knew that a hot shower was in order. First, I meticulously brushed my teeth, complete with several rinses and floss. That would ease up the pain, and better prepare my body for a delicious sleep and stretching in the morning. As I massaged the goat's milk lotion lovingly between my toes and up my calves, knees, and thighs after my shower I realized that I had finally achieved the ease of healing hardship.

The story I have shared is just one example of how somatic our emotions are. Before we can even say a word it's all in our body. It's been that way since the beginning of our lives and always will be. Techniques and treatments like reiki, acupuncture, and cupping can help us release long-term bottled up emotions. Regular exercise is also beneficial because it sets the tone for a process of regular optimum release and healthy coping in difficult situations.

The process of emotional release starts with our decision to self-nurture but sometimes we can't do it alone. That's why I wrote this book. I want to give you every tool possible so that you can:

- Achieve complete emotional healing
- Learn why releasing dark and difficult emotions is important for physical, emotional and spiritual wellness
- Have a complete system to guide you so that you can transform your heart and mind

Throughout **Detached Love: Transforming Your Heart So That You Can Transform Your Mind** we will dive deep into the inner and outer geography of our emotions. You'll discover where they live in the body and how to receive them as well as how you can release and express both negative and positive emotions. You'll learn about the heart cycles, disease and how we can heal our own bodies using our emotions as a power source. You'll also learn how to restructure our mindset to pay attention to alert of an oncoming trigger, how to refresh your inner and outer world, and who is worthy of being in your close circle of friends and gets the privilege of highly influencing you. By knowing YOUR own values and knowing how to honor them, you will naturally convey that message to those around you. Putting everyone and everything before ourselves out of duty is the expected and accepted thing to do. We do it because complying makes us good people and because we want to belong. Belonging is a very human desire. We all want to be loved and have a place in the world but when the need for belonging is combined with our desire to make our missions and our visions to change the world a reality we often begin to feel that our choices are limited. You will find that the people who truly belong in your world will appreciate the true you and those who don't will leave. That will free you to be yourself and to continue to attract the people who deserve you.

You may now find what I am proposing hard to believe. You may not even realize that you are accepting other people's projections or have excused disrespectful behavior in those closest to you for a variety of reasons. Often females are brought up to be caretakers and males to be providers. At the beginning, when we're four or five years old, we feel seen and adored. However, as we become teenagers, life becomes a drag. By then we have started to know the world a little and realize that we have "needs" which are quickly squashed by the validation we used to enjoy. Depending on our experience of life, now we see it as: judgement, shaming, categorizing and guilting. Instead of speaking up we shut down our desires, or numb our emotions or avoid them all together. In the end, all roads lead to resentment.

On a physical level, this resentment becomes joint pain. If we are athletes this means we are more susceptible to injury. Perhaps we may have various 'minor' forms of inflammation or migraines. We are easily susceptible to chest colds or other 'seasonal' viral infections. On a more severe level and after years, you may develop an autoimmune disease, have miscarriages or be completely infertile, develop high blood pressure or diabetes, have adrenal fatigue or some other thyroid issue.

On an emotional level numbing, avoidance or ignoring feelings can result in making the choice to engage in damaging activities like over exercising, over working, or being an overachiever, or to stay in socially acceptable relationships which may actually be toxic. A common example of this is marrying the "perfect catch" and existing in a living hell. The common thread is all of these seem to be desirable choices on the surface they are damaging long term. More obvious damaging choices are overeating, oversleeping, binge watching, binge drinking, excessive gaming or social media.

When the suffering starts we begin to operate on autopilot. We are not okay but always say that we're fine because it's better to not let others worry. While you are not consciously identifying whether we are in fight, flight or freeze, most often if you are numb, you are in freeze.

> If this sounds familiar, ask yourself:
> Is this living or existing?
> Do you really know your purpose?
> Who are you living for and how is that working for you?

Two miscarriages, postpartum depression, juggling a family and a high pressure career caused me to ask myself these very same questions. My quest to find the answers led me to leave my corporate job as a controller for an IT start-up. I began to study and practice Unani Tibb, a form of traditional Islamic Medicine that incorporates elements of ancient traditions including the Greek humours, Chinese Medicine and may appear similar to Ayurveda. I studied and practiced Essentrics ™, a fitness program that promotes movement and provides strength and greater mobility and I earned a certificate in sports nutrition and learned other ancient healing herbal techniques and breathing practices.

I homeschooled my six children and thrived as a part of the homeschooling community where I coordinated activities, ran Girl Scout and Boy Scout troops, and created deep connections with my children. As I achieved greater emotional healing I also discovered more of my purpose. I began to pour the knowledge I had gained from over 25 years of studying and practicing herbal medicine, fitness, and emotional healing into others. I coached women and taught them how to nurture themselves and wrote <u>The Guide How to Get Started with Workout Around My Day.</u>

<u>America's Leading Ladies: who positively impact the world, 1 Habit for Success SmartFem Edition,</u> and <u>The Art of Unlearning Volume 2</u>, the three books I've co-authored, became bestsellers and I had the wonderful experience of contributing to the best-selling book <u>America's Leading Ladies </u>where Oprah Winfrey also shared her words of wisdom.

In 2019, I was named the ACHI Magazine Volunteer of the Year, I became a LinkedIn Global Goodwill Ambassador and was voted Best Podcast Host of the Year in the United Kingdom by Powerhouse Global for my podcast The Free to Be Show. In 2020, I was named an Ambassador of Peace by the Institute of Peace and Development, finalist for the Sexy Brilliant Award, finalist for Top Influencer of 2020 by the Women's Success Conference, inducted into the Global Literary Library of Female Authors and showed up powerfully in the diversity, equity and inclusion space. I was invited to speak at Amplify DEI, on mothers in the workplace and L& D Cares growth Summit on Allyship and Transforming by Being.

In my work as an Emotions Opener and Transformation Strategist, I have shown women how to use their darkest and most difficult emotions to show up in their lives powerfully. Through my story and the stories of women I've worked with, you'll see how we often love in complete attachment, drain ourselves of the same, and experience illness and negative emotions that hold us back. You will also see how to release those damaging negative emotions and detach from the need to do what is accepted and expected to find healing we so desperately need.

In this book, you'll learn how to disentangle and still love. I will teach you how to transform your heart so that you can transform your mind using Replenish Me ™, my complete system of self-nurturing built on nutritional, fitness, scientific and spiritual practices. In step one, Release, you learn how to show yourself compassion and how to forgive yourself. Step two, Restructure, shows you how to build habits that support you physically and mentally. Refresh, step three, is all about creating firm boundaries in your relationships and the final step, Rebirth, shows you how to embody it all and to radiate and attract what you desire in your life. In each chapter, you'll receive the steps to achieve emotional release along with activities and practical ways to use them in your daily life sprinkling in the success stories of myself and others to help guide you through this life-changing process. And finally you'll learn how you can show up in the world as the powerful being you're meant to be in a full rebirth!

Here's to your healing! Let it begin :)

CHAPTER 1

CHOOSE LOVE OVER ANGER

Quote:

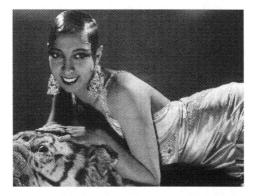

"I did take the blows [of life], but I took them with my chin up,
in dignity, because I so profoundly love and respect humanity."
~ Josephine Baker

Main idea: The main idea is to make people aware of where the emotions live in the body and clues in ailments or aches and pains. I will touch on how our words create that reality.

Anecdote:

Have you ever told someone a story about something you have experienced and then started feeling it deeply and impactfully in your body? Did it feel good? Did it feel like release or reliving? There's always this push for us to talk out things we want to let go of, however, we can relive those things by giving words to them and, the fact is, even when we talk it out some of those negative emotions are still left trapped inside of us.

I believe that if you feel your words as you think of them instead of speaking them aloud, they move out of your body. Instead of giving the negative energy of what you have experienced to someone else by giving them all of the juicy details, you can leave it and let it go back out into the ether. You can also free yourself and release the trauma that lives inside of you with physical activity. This may include movement, screams, yells, and tears. Sometimes just being open to releasing your trauma, your body will take over for your body like with PTSD or grief. I have experienced waking in the night to the sound of my own crying. Startled that it was me, I calmed myself through breathing and simple joint massage. If your trauma is physical you have to do something physical to extract it. Rhythmic movement or shaking to skin covered drums in its simplest form is a way to process your thoughts and feelings. In this case, in my workshops I invite women to release regression through their hips with a series of movements and dance. I also use the vibration of your own voice, sounds, rhythm and frequencies. When we are intentional and strategic with it, we can heal past trauma. For example, hip and low back pain has been a recurring theme for me. Through practicing pilates after my second pregnancy I found out that much of my problem was that my psoas was contracted. This is a 16 in long muscle which lives from your rib cage to the inner thigh, pelvis and ball and socket hip joint. This muscle is also very sensitive to our emotions especially when we are afraid. So if you suffer from sciatica pain or have lower back complaints, dig a little deeper into the original emotional trauma or ongoing story that you allow to live in your body.

In her book <u>The Universe Is a Green Dragon</u> physicist Dr. Briane Swimme says, "We need to crawl and climb and run if we are to develop our intellectual, emotional, and spiritual capacities...we tend to think of exercise as losing weight, as trimming off the fat. But to exercise is to enable the body to remember its past, so that it can stretch out with all its intertwined powers of being and thought and reflection." Wellness educator Joanne Cannon defines being physically fit as "the ability to meet the physical demands of one's day, plus one emergency"

Information: Why release is important

While you may be aware of the effects toxins from our environment and in food have on your bodies, you may not have the same awareness of the impact of negative energy and emotions. There are peptides that travel all through our higher brain centers including the frontal cortex which is more of a bliss center rather than a fight or flight center and tightly connected to our emotions as well as decision making. When we have negative thoughts, they send direct messages to the immune system to be on alert for an attack but it is a false alert as there are no actual bacteria or viruses to fight only thoughts. Inflammation is the accumulated ammunition of those messages over years and present in the form of regular colds or aches on the low end and adrenal fatigue, arthritis and cancer on the high end. So as the negative thoughts come, we must release them daily and if possible in the moment to prevent our bodies from storing ammunition to create disease. In her collaborative study with Bill Farrar from the Cancer Institute and Michael from the Dental Institute, Dr. Candace Pert, a psycho immunologist, discovered that the same receptors in the peptides exist on immune cells. They researched IL-1, the polypeptide "that mediate the inflammatory reactions caused by injury, trauma, or activated by the immune system... It causes fever, activates T-cells, induces sleep, and puts the body in a generally healing state of being allowing it to mobilize its energy reserves to fight pathogenic intruders with maxim efficiency." (p.163 Molecules of Emotions, Candace Pert) In the Tibb tradition release is called creating a healing crisis which is achieved through fasting. While intermittent fasting is similar to Islamic fasting, intention, also known as mindset, surrounding an action drives the outcome. Islamic fasting is more about a spiritual cleansing which benefits the body by extracting toxins. Intermittent fasting focuses only on the benefits of the body and may not release the deeper emotional and energetic toxins. In my life, during times of grief like the story I opened with in the introduction, letting go of a toxic friendship, I felt this happening in my body.

Where negative emotions live in the body

As I previously mentioned, negative emotions live in our cells so they are literally everywhere in our body. Most often they will set up residence in the joints and the lymphatic system. These are the places which limit mobility and energetic flow in the body. For women more particularly they get trapped in our fat cells and you will have swelling in the thighs, belly, hips, buttocks, arms and even your breast. In the chapter on Showing Up Powerfully, I will dive deeply into a full body resolution for this. Briefly, I will share with you now that it is a blend of taking back ownership of your sexual story, body and sexuality as a whole going forward. Self-pleasure helps you to explore your body in a new way to better understand what you truly enjoy and desire. You can tie your thoughts, words, places you touch without the interference of another and imagine that someone else is involved all the while. It is literally restructuring the muscle and fat cell memory. This is so powerful to practice whether in a relationship or not. It will take intercourse to an entirely different level.

How trapped negative emotions cause harm

These trapped emotions cause us aches and pains which we ignore or self-medicate with prescription painkillers, excessive sugar, excessive behaviors, legal drugs like alcohol or illegal drugs when we need something stronger to avoid, ignore and deny our emotions. Even if we don't self-medicate, the emotional toxins lower our cellular function and make us less productive. Fibroids, ovarian cancer, breast cancer, aneurysms, diabetes, lymphatic and adrenal conditions are some common disorders that occur as a result.

How we perceive release negatively

So many times I hear that you must be the strong Black woman and "suck it up" or "put on your big girl panties", etc. all variations of fight, flight or freeze when it comes to acknowledging, accepting your emotions to begin with and then release them. Here I am highlighting Black women because I am one and our collective pain is invisible. What makes it invisible is that it is not spoken about although studied and analyzed deeply and often used against us. What reinforces that invisibility is how Black women accept those projections in silence. We do it because we are frozen from witnessing how our mothers and grandmothers have been treated. We are frozen because we have been told, showed, voted against, and institutionalized to believe that we don't matter. In my journey, I have rebelled ranging from passive aggressive, out right rage and depression. What I have learned in Unani Tibb is to extract toxins like negative emotions, we create a healing crisis through "cooking" the body i.e. fever or fasting. Yes, fevers are not easy however when you understand their purpose, you welcome the process without resistance. This has helped me to heal and process decisions surrounding injustices like police brutality against Black women, as reasons to keep doing my work in accessing my darkest emotions to show up powerfully. It helps me to not dishonor my body in the process and use my emotions as weapons against it. Rather I have enhanced and expanded my Replenish Me ™ process to embody more body wisdom to release. Is it easier to hold it in and die? Let's explore some ways to turn this around.

Application: Ways release can be achieved

When I began researching ways to release my own grief, postpartum depression, depression and frustration I discovered there are many schools of thought and they all lead to the same answers. Most commonly spoken about are the Ayurvedic Chakra System, scientific research, and the new buzzword, Emotional Intelligence, but there are many others including tasawif commonly known as Sufism. To keep things simple, I chose the ones that worked best for me and my clients then combined what I learned with my decades long studies of nutrition, fitness, mindfulness, Islamic Traditional Medicine or Unani Tibb and created my own system for emotional release with my own values.

As I did my research and discovery, I learned we store many of the negative things we experience in our bodies without even knowing it. They literally become muscle memories and chemical imbalances. An example of ailments associated with emotions are "women with episodic urinary symptoms often find that the episodes are accompanied by anger or feeling 'pissed off'" and can be the body's way of releasing anger." (Women's Bodies, Women's Wisdom, Dr. Christiane Northrup p. 261). Energetically when you are unwilling to cope in a healthy way, set healthy boundaries and lack courage surrounding the negative aspects of unhealthy relationships in your life you will have chronic, vulvar, vaginal and urinary tract problems. Chronic stress and specific attitudes about sex can even change the blood flow to the cervical region. The best cure is love, forgiveness and good nutrition to overcome and reproductive abnormality or whether your DNA is weakened or strengthened.

Our reproductive organs are suspended in muscle and fat cells. In the fluid part of these cells special structures called mitochondria create fuel from the foods we eat providing the energy required for specific and vital activities, and they help our bodies grow and detoxify. Mitochondria are also found in abundance in muscle, fat, and liver cells. This is very important because these are the places in the body which take the brunt of our emotional trauma.

Mitochondria have their own DNA and create their own proteins, however unlike regular DNA is not self-repairing. For example, in women this may look like irregular menstrual cycles, fibroids, or other reproductive issues. Irregular periods may occur during the first eighteen months after a girl begins her menstrual cycle as her body becomes accustomed to menstruation, but if they persist throughout the first five years of puberty they may be a sign of deeper emotional issues. If these issues are dealt with correctly more serious reproductive disorders and ailments can be prevented.

The following diagrams show where we hold energy in our body, how our emotions impact us, and list the ailments that result when negative emotions go unaddressed for an extended period of time. As you can see in the following diagram, our body has different energy centers called chakras.

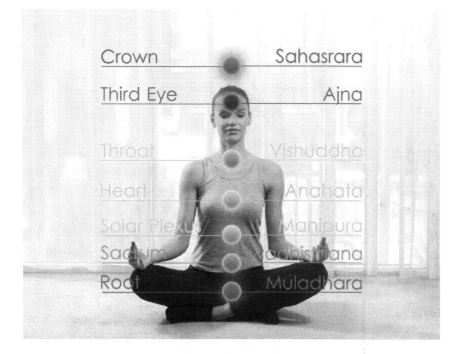

The chakras are said to be seven energy centers in the body where each chakra relates to a specific gland in the endocrine system. They all connect and spiral up fueled by sexual energy at the root. Most people express sexual energy through sexual activity which kills it. The more productive option is to allow it to flow upward to the crown.

1. Root - reproductive and life force
2. Sacral - adrenal glands

3. Solar plexus - willpower
4. Heart
5. Throat - Thyroid gland
6. Third eye - Brain
7. Crown - pituitary gland

In Islam, for example, men and women are encouraged to fast to positively channel that energy especially when not married. It is also a protection from succumbing to your lower self, depression, idleness, worry and overthinking. I will dive more into sexual energy and fasting in a later chapter. The idea to embrace in this chapter is that sexual energy is a creative life force of its own. Focusing on the source of the energy (Divine power/ Allah/Jesus, etc.), keeps you healthy, productive, in service to your purpose and away from your ego. It helps you to attain true compassion. The emotions are a bridge between the physical and spiritual worlds and have a map in our body. For example, the psoas muscle covers the area where anger, fear, love, passion, rejection live. Disappointment lives in our kidneys, grief in our thighs, our expectation of loving support and financial support in our hips. When we release the expectations from others, we can channel that energy upward into ourselves to accept our own love and connect with the blessings that God has for us. Otherwise we block ourselves in fear and anger for who did not offer, provide or help. Free yourself to be a vessel for the Divine to offer, provide and guide. It will allow us simple pleasures like actually receiving a compliment for face value. That is true self-compassion.

Welcoming that new worldview is self-forgiveness. Instead of following the human pattern of shaming, blaming and guilting ourselves for not being more open to God's wisdom or receiving His abundance, you unlock that part of yourself that says, "it's okay you did the best you could with the information and knowledge you had at the time. Offer yourself grace and mercy and evolve."

When you continue to practice these two steps over and over and over, that's when your self- belief muscle can take over and if you practice it enough you show up in full self-trust. One woman told me "Rebirthing is no joke sis. Feels like I went through an explosion of the soul with a massive blast from the past. It's been a crucial 6 weeks of intense 'labour pain"

I replied, "...rebirth on a personal level is a refinement of who we are and just like bringing a child into the world is a process. Your inner and outer self have to be in harmony and push together in order for gravity to take over and allow that portal between worlds to open."

Self-compassion is being very clear on your values and honoring them. This allows you to separate from what's expected and accepted in your culture, household and family.

We are taught to attach love to an object. The truth is the tether between you and love starts at the source...the Creator of all. Imagine an invisible thread between you and values and anything which outweighs that thread doesn't get a ride. As you grow and evolve it will feel new and strange. Loving yourself and creating your own sense of belonging without judgement takes self-forgiveness. Self-forgiveness is giving yourself grace for growing, evolving and blossoming. Ask yourself the following questions: Have you grown, evolved and moved on? Or are you harboring Ill-feelings towards yourself? Free yourself! Those were learning opportunities! Do you see the lesson? Are you benefiting from the wisdom? Forgive, let it be and remember it all led to this present moment. Self -belief is showing up as your true self because that's the BEST YOU! Where is your focus? Is it learning or applying what you've learned with your unique spin? Imagination is our filter for processing information. Otherwise the knowledge is just a pool of abstract concepts. Aim higher and restructure your mind by activating your imagination. Through the process of releasing thoughts and habits with self-compassion and self-forgiveness and completing the process with self-belief, you can reprogram your life with Replenish Me ™!

Action Steps

Release exercise: Are you ready for a reset?

It all starts with release. Feel into your body with movement deep in the hips, waist and torso. Imagine yourself as a belly dancer and move in a circular and alternating spiral motion. Give yourself up to the movement. It may help to listen to a freeing song like Angelique Kidjo's "Bahia". Close your eyes and move your hips to the slow rhythm. Experiment with circles and spirals in your hips and torso. Just feel, do and be.

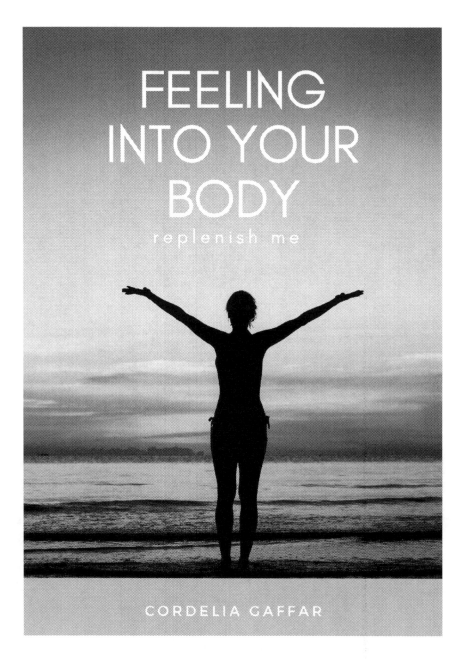

FEELING
INTO YOUR
BODY
replenish me

CORDELIA GAFFAR

FEELING IT INTO YOUR BODY

self expression

receiving love, compassion

willpower, passion

emotional and financial support

sexual energy and belief to do anything

NEGATIVE EMOTIONS IN YOUR BODY

despair, grief

other people's burdens

fear, anger

repression, abandonment

shame and guilt

frustration

NEGATIVE EMOTIONS

=

DOWNWARD EMOTIONAL FLOW

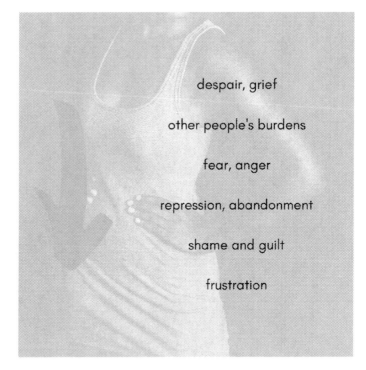

despair, grief

other people's burdens

fear, anger

repression, abandonment

shame and guilt

frustration

WHAT'S THE STORY YOU HAVE BEEN CARRYING?

In the space below, capture your guilt, shame, judgement or any other story you have been carrying since your childhood.

REFLECTION

Reflect on how your story has played out for you so far.
Describe below how you have been showing up and whether it's true.
Then describe how you can change or rewrite it.

_____

_____

_____

_____

_____

_____

_____

_____

_____

_____

_____

_____

_____

_____

_____

_____

_____

_____

_____

_____

CREATING YOUR MAP-BRAIN DUMP

Using what you have written so far, perform a brain-dump below, on your top three desires to turn your life around.

CORDELIA GAFFAR | ©2020

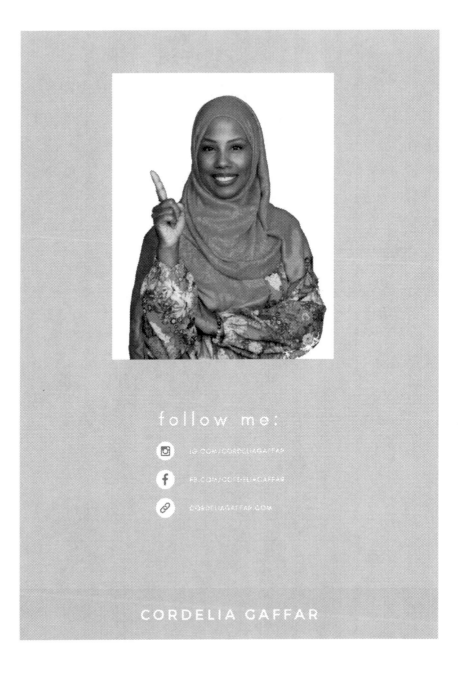

CHAPTER 2

RELEASE

Quote:
"Surrender to receive that's how you are liberated"
- Cordelia Gaffar

Main idea: Release - What is expected and accepted. Release the need to accept others projections.

Anecdote:

I was asked to explain the above quote on the Susan Brender Show. I said that," When you detach from the outcome or expectation, you open your heart to receiving the blessing. That liberates you because now you are grateful for it." Receiving and gratitude become a flow instead of a dam blocked by our self-doubt or desperation. For so many years I walked without talking. Now I find myself in a space where I am talking for all of the years I have not. Some days, I see myself as someone else who is allowing the catch up and not as someone who is talking about my current walk. In my mind, this was not meant to be a riddle but a stream of consciousness so stay with me. I found that my mind can liberate or elevate me if I allow. I got curious and asked myself: Are you walking your talk? Or just talking without moving? Or just moving? I started to imagine what it would feel like if I nourished my dreams, focused on nurturing my body and speaking freely. I imagined breaking free so that I offer myself what I require to breathe freely. I had to take my mind there because even in a home filled with people, my husband and children, I felt that I had no one to share my vision with. I chose to create an opportunity to show myself some compassion. I knew it was not a time to let self- doubt takeover. I understand sometimes people cannot see me because of a difference in worldview and vision or it is a catalyst. It's about your gift not their opinions. I had to replenish with love. I had to Release the need for their acceptance and approval. My hips were on freeze so I welcomed soca back into my life to free them. I say it best in this poem:

> Have you ever tried it?
> That's what it's like to Replenish...intrigued?
> Step into my world where we explore, examine and re-establish the "norm"
> Want your mind to shush?
> Want to feel again?
> Want to see yourself loving your perfectly imperfect form?
> It's not a brain strain
> It's simply a bounce into the little embrace of self-compassion
> Let me show the way....
> That's what it's like to Replenish...piqued?
> Step into my world where we dip, dive and climb out of the expected
> Want your heart to beat?
> Want clarity again?
> Want to stop yourself from being misdirected?
> It's quite plain
> Let's be on our way, you and I together

Information:

One tool I use to help my clients manage their daily vibration is by having a theme for each day. Below I will define the meaning for each day. In the next section, create your own objective using the daily themes. And yes they are hashtags because everything is a hashtag these days. It helps to keep you accountable and post in the Facebook group. I will share a sample post that I've posted in my group to provoke thought for each activity.

The Daily Themes
Sweet Talk ™ Sunday
Mindfull Monday
Tools and Fuel Tuesday
What I Desire Wednesday
Terrific Thursday
Freeing Friday
Self-Nurturing Saturday

Definitions and Application:

Sweet Talk Sunday is a great way to start the week by selecting a word to guide you. During the writing of this book, I chose to plan my words ahead of time through acronyms. Sometimes, I knew the words and sometimes I had place holders. Here's an example:

J - Joy
O - Opportunity/ Opulence
Y - You
F - Freedom
U - Unleash
L - Love

Notice I had two words for the letter **O**. Depending on your heart's desire or gravity you will feel a pull towards one word or the other. The main thing is to be present in every moment to know what you require for emotional stability.

Mind Full Monday is stepping back and taking a deeper look at things you may allow to happen or do on autopilot. For example, you may dismiss your spouse by always leaving the closet door open or yell at him for doing it although you deeply feel that it is an accident waiting to happen and disrespectful of your daily request. This was a major issue for me for many years. My husband would leave the closet door open and I would mention it to him. He would close the door while I am looking. Somehow when I wake up in the night, I run into the door. Yes, on the surface it's not a big deal but in the end I saw evidence of how I let "the little things slide" throughout our life.

Mindfull Monday is about being aware of the "mini-patterns" in your life that individually are not a big deal but collectively make your life miserable. I used to hate the quote, "the way you do one thing is the way you do all things". When I took a personal inventory it was because it hit home. As I observed my patterns of behavior and truly became a student of myself, I saw how I was great at not eating junk food until I had a fight with my husband, the kids had a full mutiny on homeschooling or soccer games scheduled shifted last minute. Suddenly I was at the mercy of others. I had lost control. My sleep would suffer from my much needed 7 hours plus afternoon nap to 3-4 heavily interrupted hours. That caused me to think negatively, be evil and speak more bad things into reality and on a deeper level get triggered from "old stuff". In this sleep deprived state my mind could not function and went straight into survival/ adrenaline mode. When I realized what was happening, I made a conscious effort to stop and allow the emotional overwhelm to wash over me and be grounded as it passed. What my children saw was me completely frozen, emotionless, expressionless. They fought, laughed and I gave up the battle of my triggers and emotions. I would stare at the sky or grass or something in nature to calm myself. Sometimes if it was really bad, I would also massage essential oils on my finger joints.

Tools and Fuel Tuesday is about using tools you have access to to resolve issues that you may let slide. Going back to the issue in Mindfull Monday, there may be a communication tool that you are using at work that would be effective with resolving the underlying issues with your spouse above and beyond closing the closet door.

Fuel is related to how to eat or exercise to support you for the day. I use this to pay attention to my habits. Sometimes, I realize that I'm feeling super tired all of the time. So I journal what I'm eating, how much I'm sleeping nightly, how much I'm moving daily. If I discover that I'm sleeping 7 hours a night and going to bed at decent hours, eating a balanced diet and not slipping into daily patterns of excessive candy, coffee, savory, etc but not moving much, I will set my alarm to move for 10 minutes before breakfast, lunch and dinner or 5 minutes at the end of every waking hour.

What I Desire Wednesday is about recognizing and honoring what you truly desire to exist in your life. The above is a great example of exploring that if you have never tried.

Terrific Thursday is knowing that we can set the tone of the day just by choosing our own vibration. Yes it really is that simple. Deciding that today is the perfect day to...is within your reach.

Freeing Friday is about freeing yourself from others expectations.

Self-Nurturing Saturday is lovingly lean into your day, listen for your breath, step gently and with purpose and be present

Tips and Activities:

Sunday Activity: Create an acronym for the next month with corresponding words.

Instructions: The first word you choose of course would stand for the current week leaving flexibility for all others. Here's how it works. Think of a simple phrase that applies to what is the most desired outcome in your heart. For me it was, ***Let it go!*** That time I was really struggling to make a life changing decision and had financial, emotional and marital problems all at once. Despite my laissez faire disposition, I was still quite controlling and guarded.

Coming up with Sweet Talk ™ Sunday words has to be planned. While I believe in spontaneity and being inspired, you must control the boat. Leading up to my trip to London, I created an acronym which gave me structure and freedom all in one. In other words, I already knew that my word for each week would be limited by the beginning letter but what the word would be was left to my needs, experiences or inspiration that week. Yes of course, I picked a word for each letter simply as a placeholder.

Monday Activity: In keeping with your word of the week, how can you see the pattern, pause and reflect its deeper meaning for you, discern your emotions surrounding it and find a resolution for it? Where do our thoughts come from?

- Triggers from our subconscious
- Feelings that we hold in our passion and heart center
- Unknown inspiration
- Our DNA

Tuesday Activity:

Okay, maybe it wasn't a divorce it could have been a never-ending toxic relationship or marriage

WHATEVER It was! It's not serving you anymore so leave it!

I'm not going to say that you deserve better.

I'm not going to give you advice. But for once can you just stop and listen to the sound of your own heart beating? If you close your eyes and breathe deeply you may even hear it speak to you…

"That shaming and judging voice doesn't belong to you…the truth is…let's do it!…stop waiting!"

Can you hear that?

I know right? Probably have heard it many times before but ignored it because everyone else's voice was louder.

Or probably because you denied it...or felt guilty for even acknowledging it

So let's refuel with strengthening thoughts:

I am strong because I love with all of my heart

I am wise because I know what I need

I am ...(this one's for you to workout)

Wednesday Activity: After reading the post below, make a list of what you truly desire so that you can vibrate at your highest in love with yourself.

As Lenny Kravitz says, "We got to let love rule!"

That love has to begin within and we teach others how to love us by setting clear boundaries that keep us replenished.

So on What I Desire Wednesday reflect on what you need to keep you centered, sane, sleeping and eating on time.

How can you delegate?

Who needs to know this?

What is it that needs to come off your plate?

These questions although simple may be difficult to answer if you have spent most of your life giving to others or are very emotionally guarded.

Freeing Friday: Free Yourself to Feed Yourself

Friday Activity:

It's shocking to me how many women don't know how to take care of their bodies. Yes, I just said that!

I can't tell you how many times I've heard, "I eat well." While I watch them eat processed meats or too much food at the wrong time during the day or drinking caffeine when their body clearly is asking for water or actual food.

Even more intriguing is when I will hear, "I'm not a breakfast person. I eat when my body is hungry". Then I ask, "how do you know when your stomach is hungry?"

The answer is always, "my stomach makes noise"

Even worse, I know several recent cases of women my age being admitted to the hospital for several weeks due to extreme anemia, low blood volume, and complete malnutrition. How does that even happen in the first world?

Wake up women!

You don't understand the signs your body is sending you. You have the same relationship with your body that you have with everyone else in your life except worse! Listen to me.

I'm not calling you out for shock value, this is serious. This hospital check in was just a warning sign. Next time, you might be dead!

It's time that you become a true observer of the alerts, subtle messages and whispers your body sends you all day long. The gentle kiss in the morning with your breath that says, "Wake up girl" ever so softly. Maybe the yawn, that prompts you for a glass of water which you answer with a cappuccino or perhaps a Red Bull. The pre-rumble of your digestive tract after the water or coffee that says, time for food which you respond to with a cookie or continuous pieces of candy or maybe nothing. Then the loud growl that demands food which you satiate with something inadequate like a piece of gluten free vegan pizza or salad with too much salad dressing instead of a high quality meal fit for a queen.

Does any of this sound familiar?

I know we think that we are eating "well" when we have the trending gluten-free vegan bullsh*t or salad doused with high calorie dressing or even the low quality vinaigrette. But I'm here to tell you that when you are working the hardest, thinking the most and out there changing the world, that's when your body requires the most food in the form of high quality nutrition.

During my last trip in London, one of my colleagues and I went to lunch. She said," you can eat girl and you're so tiny!" I responded, "it's because I eat so much that I'm tiny because I give my body what it needs when it needs it and sometimes even before."

When we don't allow the constant starvation cycles to set in is when we are nourished. The more you eat during your working hours or before, the less you'll eat when you are sitting idle. It's the idle, mindless eating that weighs us down. That weight is mostly mentally in the end because the brain is overburdened from having to run the show on empty which has the hormones stattered and the stomach hoping for some type of acknowledgment that comes too late.

Saturday Activity: Liberate your mind with the timelessness of time!

This time last week, I was helping to set up and attend this beautiful event and receive my first international award. This weekend I am pouring back into my body with rest, nourishing food and connecting with my children. All powerful ways to be replenished in your body. Now that you have gone through the daily themes and complete with activities, what have you released? What have you learned about yourself? Who would you be or how your life would have been different if you chose a higher vibration a decade ago? What if you were gifted a better chance at something you lost? Everything is still there waiting for you, receptive to your every whim and readily available. All you have to do is show up and say yes. Then every time you say yes, more doors open for you not just concerning those things but everything in your life.

Sweet Talk ™ receives abundance and pour into yourself abundantly open to receiving, especially when you are intentional and specific with your request.

You may have seen my pictures with my daughters this weekend. It was such a pleasure to have them with me as I was recognized by my peers for Volunteer of the Year by ACHI magazine. They see me working daily via video calls and on my phone on the way to their various activities. While they love and support me, I notice that they are doing the same with their friends and my ways are becoming their ways. They were tickled to see me up on stage as they took pictures and recorded my brief acceptance speech with my youngest daughter by my side.

She was so looking forward to speaking on stage and so I brought her with me. Even remembering sharing that moment with all of them fills me with joy now. This weekend, I am up for another award at SpeakerCon, the brainchild of Cheryl Wood. I won't be able to bring them with me but at least, I won't be in London...where I started the month of receiving awards :)

I'm sharing all this to say, "be receptive to abundance"! When we are intentional and specific with our aims, it will come. Be open to recognizing and receiving it. Don't keep your head down and let it pass by you or have your guard up in suspicion. Stand tall and welcoming as it embraces you and envelopes you in pure joy. Then share it with those closest to you, for me my daughters and sons :)...allow that joy to replenish you and your purpose so that you continue to powerfully impact the world! That can be a nap, a walk or a delicious meal. It could be reading a book or listening to a podcast or maybe just staring at a wall whatever it is connected with your inner wisdom and strength.

CHAPTER 3

WHAT YOU CARRY ON YOUR SHOULDERS AND KNOWING YOUR VALUES

Quote: "When someone asks you why you choose the way you do, the answer is: 'Because that's what I chose'. ~ Cordelia Gaffar

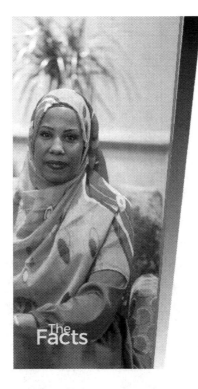

When someone ask you why you choose the way you do, the answer is :

"Because that's what I chose"

~ Cordelia Gaffar

Main Idea: Who are we living for and why does it seem like life is so heavy? This is the hunch in your shoulders and the weight on your neck. It affects your breathing and your mindset heavily.

Anecdote:

Changing your inner voice is like leaving a toxic relationship. It is a disentangling that may seem insurmountable. Have you ever had a chest cold? You know how it can feel like all of the crying that you never allowed all at one time in your chest? Your lungs are heavy with the clouds of inflammation. Your throat eeks out a cup full of mucus that leave tread marks and feel like the scratch of evil. You strive just to breathe without really breathing, escape without ever leaving and cry without tears really ever falling from your eyes...replenish Me? I thought to myself, 'Am I lying to everyone? Most importantly am I lying to myself?' During the time that I am writing this book, I am being tested in every relationship. Because this is my story and the entanglement of people close to me are immense, I will share the outer layers of my personal situation in this chapter and have enlisted some friends to share their full stories of overwhelm to overflow. You can probably relate to things going wrong as being a heaviness on your soul. So what am I doing in each of these difficult moments I am being gifted now? Where do I begin a sustainable way to reprogram my inner voice? Yes, I am taking my own advice and choosing only what honors me. I pause kindly for the cause to free myself of others' expectations. Up until now, I have always struggled with doing what was expected and when I did it, performed very robotically. Silently I feel life is escaping with each breath, each expected choice, each bite of mindless eating Sweet Tarts or drinking a cappuccino, each extra numbing moment exercising excessively or each moment ignoring myself. Before Covid -19, in times like these, I found my way back by taking the leap and going on a retreat. That's where my true healing began. So I created a virtual retreat with a colleague. I can remember when I used to laugh at women who swore by the benefits of traveling to go on retreat. I used to think, *'how can running away from your problems possibly help you?'* But having made a practice of taking at least one retreat per year for the last three, I now know that it is so very necessary to be away from the very elements of your life that exclude you from yourself. Yes, you read that right. I was living my life as a cog in a wheel not as an essential part of the engine. That's why I wanted to get away so that I could see myself and acknowledge my humanness and importance. So going on retreat helps you to be an active member in your life. The act of leaving everything you know to explore a new place opens a different part of your brain. Whether you intend to or not, it will even open a different part of your heart. With that opening I gave myself freely to having a transformative experience in a safe space with like hearts and off load what I carry on my shoulders.

You may wonder how I replicated that virtually, which I will share more that below. Here's a part of my healing in poetry:

Who are you really?

Are you the person you think you are? How did you become the way you are now?

This is self-reflection piece,

A new direction reach

In the moment, you let it go or pass it until next time

But why?

Who are you really?

Are you that silly, little girl who loved to play and was shut down

Are you the frolicking young professional all over town

Now that you have "matured" who have you come to be?

Did you make you or did they make you see

That the you that you are is not worthy

Did you choose to run and swerve into here

The here that is neither here nor there

The here that has you running everywhere

And still you neither know or see

The you that is really you

Or the one you wish to be

So who are you really?

Have you any idea?

Has it crossed your mind lately

Have you given up who you are innately

For a shell of who you could be

Would you be greatly

Surprised to find you again just by taking a moment to pour back within

Rather than to run your knuckles bare and your heart to despair

Are you open to repair the damage before it's insurmountable

Or are you already there?

Who are you really?

Willing to start and be a part of your healing

Dealing with all the things that aren't even yours

Just makes life to be one huge list of chores

What if you could work in a reframe and retrain you heart

Transform your brain

Replenish yourself and begin again?

Would you, could you be willing to try?

It is easy, it is easy as pie

Starting to feel jiggly inside?

Are you ready to say, 'I am open and no longer willing to hide!'

Information:

What is the weight that you carry on your shoulders? It's the energy and expectations of your partner, boss, children, parents and the list goes on. Be honest with yourself, whose energy is it which buries you alive? Take a moment to reflect. Okay, I get that you may not recognize that it's a person. Consider thinking of the words which make you feel heavy and the loudest one of your inner chatter. Are those words in alignment with what you believe or are they from someone else? It may sound something like:

'You should spend more time with your kids...'

Or

'You should make $XXX by the time you are 40...'

In fact any of the should statements, are the weight of someone else's value system and standards. Throw your shoulders back and breathe into your body. What is bubbling in your heart? Do you hear the faint voice of possibility? This voice sounds more like…

'Look how much a loving look with a smile can make up for a whole day away from your child?"

Or

'Look how far you've come despite all of the trials and tribulations…'

This is the voice of self-acceptance. That's your true inner voice. How do you make that voice louder? At the end of the day, this weight is simply words. These words we select to believe change our chemical state. Those chemicals are our emotions and become our feelings. It is all an illusion beginning with a choice.

It's simply by practicing daily. In my workshops and virtual retreats, I encourage women to think of their favorite love song and change the words as if they are singing to themselves. In other words, serenade yourself and call to your own heart with longing. You know the ones where the lovers are elevating and appreciating one another? Imagine that is your inner self singing to your outer self. Become all things replenished in your body concerning each bite you take, each movement you make and how to move those sensual parts and reignite all of your sensuality again. Become all things replenished in your soul envisioning the path you've been hiding from those closest to you for fear of rejection or incompleteness and free that intangible part of you. Become all things replenished in your emotions so that you no longer have to numb them, hide them or eat them away instead using them as your ultimate power source…How does that feel in your body?

This is a body awareness exercise. When you directly relate words to understand the various energy centers and understand what your body means with each ache or pain, you will better understand why you may get sick or feel like you've been hit by a train after a difficult conversation at work or an argument with your spouse. Connecting the words you hear and say, you will better understand the power of words. You will experience the effects of Sweet Talk ™ and how to heal yourself with it. Also allow yourself to just lean into your emotions for the full 90 seconds that they last. You will learn how to use your raw emotions as a power source and change your life. Using our emotions as a power source is our birthright as human beings. We are hard-wired to always be blissful and not miserable. For some reason we've gotten it backwards.

Here's an example of leaning into the emotion of grief. It started with a tickle in my throat which became a cry more like a whimper. At first, I ignored it as a possible grief even though it was the anniversary of my mother's death. I told myself that, 'With the temperatures dropping I'm craving warming foods.' My chest revolted and real tears started to fall. I held myself in a tight hug to regain control and to comfort myself. That's when I let myself go. I strongly smelled the aroma of thibouthiene and dal with kitchuri. These are comfort foods from different parts of my life which provided healing, love and wholeness. As I leaned into my grief, I began to strongly desire these foods. Knowing that these foods have healing qualities, I indulged. Thibouthiene is an Senegalese fish stew and no I'm not Senegalese...but in one part of my life I had a very nurturing experience after losing my mother. Kitchuri is a rice based Bangla dish I enjoyed while visiting my mother in law in Bangladesh. She also reminds me of my mother. She is loving, kind, soft -spoken and powerful, embodies what it is to be a woman of faith and a rock for her community and family. I am yearning for the warmth of my mother. My mother was my place of belonging in the world and once again I find myself lost. She would know what to do and what to say where to go. I've been praying, meditating and all the things I know to do as a transformation coach. I also know that sometimes you must be in your emotions and fully experience your feelings to rejoin the world in your full power. So just for that day, I enveloped myself in her knowing. For that week, I was more compassionate with myself.

Our brains are ever changing with each interaction...smile...hug... hibernation...hike...We choose whether it expands or withers. Body awareness and emotional wellness allow the process of neuroplasticity to take its course. Did you know that practicing a positive perspective shift can grow brain cells? Aging gracefully is all about neuroplasticity. That's what we've been talking about. It's so much deeper than reframing your perspective to the glass is always half full. It's more like the glass is always full. That's right 100% abundance thinking restructures you're neuropathways. What perspective shift will you create today? You have a choice to live full out or to shrink. Making that choice to live fully includes nourishing the brain with omega 3 and 6, calcium, magnesium, and zinc. Did you know that together these vitamins and minerals help you cope with stress? Stress coping involves, making wise choices in the moment, seeing a situation and not going into flight or fright or fight. Standing fully in your power like standing up to a wave in the ocean and swimming into the current instead of giving up. Walnuts were an essential diet staple while I was restructuring my diet to overcome postpartum depression. And yes they are high in omega 3 and 6. At the time, I chose them for the B6 or niacin levels. In fact, most nuts help regulate our hormones because of the high B vitamin content. Seeds are also a great source of omega 3&6 levels exceeding most fish. In times of stress our body experiences inflammation and a plant based diet can hydrate, detox and heal all at once. Stress is relative to you and your personality type. Sometimes we think that we are immune to stress because we have conditioned our minds to be in fight or flight mode. However, our bodies have wisdom and send us alerts by weeping or giving us aches and pains. A chronic sinus infection could be due to us consistently not speaking up or back pain could be accepting an unsupportive partner. Eating foods with omegas 3&6 and regular exercise can make life easier but tuning into the cause and eradicating it is better.

Application:

On your healing journey, you may realize that you have trouble receiving what you truly desire and also struggle to completely release what is troubling you emotionally. For example, on the physical level your left shoulder and right hip strike out when you are crumbling emotionally.

The left side is the feminine side because it is where the heart moves towards. Your shoulder is the weight of other people's burdens. Your right side is the masculine; and the hips are where you hold anger, rage, repression, powerlessness. When you don't speak up for yourself, your body cries out. Listen. According to the NIH **Pain and Disability: Clinical, Behavioral, and Public Policy Perspectives. The Anatomy and Physiology of Pain,** "Pain is a subjective experience with two complementary aspects: one is a localized sensation in a particular body part; the other is an unpleasant quality of varying severity commonly associated with behaviors directed at relieving or terminating the experience.

Pain has much in common with other sensory modalities (National Academy of Sciences, 1985). First, there are specific pain receptors. These are nerve endings, present in most body tissues, that only respond to damaging or potentially damaging stimuli. Second, the messages initiated by these noxious stimuli are transmitted by specific, identified nerves to the spinal cord." And on a metaphysical or spiritual level according to The Book of Sufi Healing(p.12), "The seat of the vegetative function - that is, the instinctive, life -sustaining work of the body- is the liver, sometimes called the Wheel of Life. All of our physical functions are cued by the functions and enzymes of the liver." Continuing onto p. 13, "Interestingly, some ailments or conditions that we have come to regard as purely emotional have their origin in physical imbalances. An example is severe anger. Psychologists would usually attribute this to a condition of the mind or emotions. But according to the Tibb system of the Persian physician Avicenna, severe anger is one of the body's most effective ways of dispelling excess moisture in the area of the heart. It is easily corrected with diet. The interaction of the three realms (or activation of the physical and mental realms by the soul realm) is carried out by means of the spirit. Many people use the words "spirit" and "soul" to mean the same thing, yet they are distinctly different and separate. The spirit activates the physical level of existence, including thought processes. The word for this ...is activated at the point of the breath."

So what does this all mean? As crazy as it sounds, sometimes the thing that could eat you alive could actually make your thrive. Seeing that your great ideas are overlooked in corporate can be frustrating but ultimately it becomes the CEO's "great idea". Sometimes, it's the unsupportive spouse who is your biggest naysayer and more than proving you can make it, you astonish with your brilliance. Your joint pain is caused by wanting more than you are receiving. When you expect from others without being specific or even verbalizing your heart's desires, it creates resentment.

As a result, you continue to accept whatever they give you and inflame your body, specifically your joints even more. What you seek is within your control. You only have to speak it into existence. Speak your truth! Our bodies cry in so many ways. Sometimes it's due to years of giving away our power through having sex with people who are not worthy of us. We have painful cramps, fibroids, cervical cancer. Sometimes through chronic STD which leads to cervical cancer. On top of the deep feeling of unworthiness that we borrow from those people we allow in our bodies, we are embarrassed to get the help we need to treat our physical expression of unworthiness and suffer physically, mentally, and emotionally until it actually kills us. Or maybe it's our stomachs which suffer through a desire to be physically appealing. We purge and don't allow our bodies the nutrition it needs because we feel good is the menu and not the words of the unworthy elements we have given power over our self-confidence. Self-acceptance and self-forgiveness are not the same thing but both are necessary for healing. You need self-acceptance to be ready to understand and embrace forgiveness. For example, you may need to accept that you are stressed at the end of the day and what happened cannot be changed. Then step into forgiving yourself because you are human and sometimes can lose your temper. Forgive yourself and look for the learning moment. Once you release what is expected and accepted behaviors in society and your community, you will be able to identify your values and create habits to honor them. This chapter is presenting the background for why knowing your values is so very important. Stop the cycle!

- Using the passion of your anger to find the learning opportunity
- Taking that learning opportunity and making it marketable
- Embracing and accepting the emotional journey of creating the life you desire

In this chapter, I'm sharing the stories of two women from very different backgrounds and cultures yet with the same physical result; ailments related to reacting to the judgement and approval of others of a woman. The women struggled with shame for being anorexic/bulimia. Her story of shame was not only one she adopted from society as a whole but her culture as well.

Carleeka

"I am a survivor of an eating disorder. I had a fear of getting fat. I could not get skinny enough. Now in the African American community this was not considered a mental illness. But I had a mental illness that started when I was in the 10th grade through adulthood. This was a secret that I kept from my family and friends. I would eat and throw up three to four times or I would not eat at all. It got to the point where I did not have to make myself throw up. It was automatic that even after eating a few crackers and sips of water I would have to vomit. This was my lifestyle.

This was my new normal, even though it was not healthy in no shape or form I had accepted this way of living. I was happy being so skinny that I could see my ribs. However, not knowing the health risks that occur during that time and later in my life. I felt like I had a sense of control. I could determine how much I wanted to weigh and eat as much or less as I wanted. Years later after recovering from having this disorder I have had so many digestive problems, such as bleeding ulcers, the lining of my stomach thinner, elevated liver enzymes as well.

At the time I have no pain in my stomach unless I get overwhelmed then my stomach will knot up and I would be in pain. I did not incur any diseases per say but I do have to be very careful of what I eat and live a stress-free life. During my healing process yes, the ailments that I have had definitely correlated to having the eating disorder. I realized they were related when I was in and out of the emergency room and being susceptible to ulcers which are extremely painful.

I have used methods of living a healthier lifestyle, using holistic remedies when and if I get ill. I am still benefiting from eating healthier and being active. When I think of Replenish Me ™, I feel that in my mind mostly. I know that if I did not change my thinking about me, life and my health that I would not be here today. The healing that has taken place in my mind and body has changed my whole life. My message to other women is to love who you are and take care of your whole self from the inside-out. Remember, by nature we are nurturing beings but we need to practice self-nurturing and self-care practices."

Now I'm sharing the story of a woman who lived for decades taking on the energy of others and it resulted in cancer and a plethora of other ailments.

Devon

"Even though a genetic disorder predisposed me for cancer, I believe stress played a huge part in this occurrence. As women, we too often take care of others before we take care of ourselves. We must remember to hear our spirit, nurture the need of self love and care, and keep ourselves healthy both physically and mentally. We cannot truly care for others, since we are natural caretakers, if we do not take care of ourselves first. I feel this spiritual pain in the core of my body, in my gut. For the longest time I have had stuck dark energy in the left side of my chest. I believe it is where I was holding all of the fear of having cancer, on that side where the tumor was discovered. It was the weirdest feeling.

At the time of diagnosis, I didn't feel anything in my body. I had been so vigilant in all of my check-ups and when I got the call it was like a kick in the gut. The mammogram was the last test of the year and I had felt so proud of myself to have kept all my scheduled appointments for surveillance. My Primary care called, and I expected it to be one of the nurses letting me know my mammogram was clear. When I answered the phone and it was my doctor, it was a hit to my stomach. It felt like someone had punched me. I knew there were two cysts that were under surveillance, but she said there was a third. I can say that dealing with fear and living with it for the next 8 years started at this time in my life.

For my entire life I have always known that I was 'lumpy and bumpy'. I have encountered tumors in my body since I was a child. Whenever I had a lump I just knew that it had to be removed. The first tumor removed was on the side of my nose when I was 13. Then there was a tumor removed in my left breast under the areola at age 14. It really became a noticeable thing, when I had a large tumor removed out of my left forearm. I never knew I had this disorder until I was 46 years old and was tested. Until then, I just always know to remove any tumor that may show up in my body. All that were removed prior to having breast cancer were benign.

In 2005 I went to the doctor to find out why I was having a hard time hearing. He ordered an MRI to determine if I had a cyst growing on the nerve in my ear. From this test it was determined I was born with a brain tumor. Later it was determined I was actually born with a rare genetic disorder called 'Cowden's Syndrome'. This is a PTEN tumor suppressor disorder which put me at risk for growing tumors throughout my body. The MRI test was the catalyst of a medical journey I have been on ever since. Since that test, I have had Thyroid removal, kidney stones, and Breast Cancer. Once I went through treatment and dealt with the after care of post cancer treatment, my life changed. The fear of cancer and what it does to the psyche was not something I expected to experience. I lived in a state of suppressed fear that I didn't realize controlled my life for 8 years. In 2016 I came off of my post cancer meds and made the decision to remove my breasts. The experience of that amputation was surreal yet freeing. The item on my body which fueled that fear I lived in was now gone. I went through reconstruction and ultimately, 2 years later, removed the implants I had put in due to inflammation in my body. It has been 12 weeks since the removal and I feel so much better. I am fighting my way back to optimum health, one step at a time. Through all of this adversity and darkness, which at times was unbearable, I face it with humor and faith. I tried to always see the light through the darkness and continue to live that way today.

I never knew anything about my genetic disorder prior to having Breast Cancer. A year after treatment, my oncologist referred me to a dermatologist and wanted me to have some bumps on my skin biopsied to insure they were nothing to worry about. During the appointment with this dermatologist, she asked me about my history. I informed her of everything and she was the doctor who picked up on my possibly having a genetic disorder. She even said 'I think you have a rare genetic disorder called Cowden's Syndrome'. Once the genetic testing was confirmed in Nov 2010, all the pieces of the puzzle seemed to fall into place. My entire history of tumors made sense. Once I looked up the symptoms and characteristics of 'Cowden's Syndrome', I basically have the majority. My skull size is larger than normal, among other things ... I could never wear cute hats like the other girls, LOL. It was a relief to finally have an answer to a lifelong experience.

This experience changed my life. I am a social individual and this experience has quieted me. People who I thought would be around as I went through this experience, weren't. I've had to learn to fend for myself but also to forgive. From a spiritual perspective, I have grown with healing the pain of abandonment from my friends, and to learn forgiveness. It was interesting to learn the fear that others feel when someone they love encounters cancer. I had friends who were afraid to be around me in fear of 'Catching' cancer. Others were fearful to see me suffer and go through treatment. It was hurtful at the time but I have learned to forgive as they do not know. Also, I had to consciously accept that should any of them walk the path that I did, I would be there for them with love and compassion.

From a physical perspective, I have adapted a general vegan dietary lifestyle and a few years ago I began using essential oils. The change has been incredible. Along with this, I have also begun exercising regularly and incorporated meditation into my daily life. It has done a world of good to be more centered spiritually and focused on the good. Don't get me wrong, I still have dark days that are very hard but I choose to focus on the light in those times and it generally always pulls me out of the darkness. My diet change, use of essential oils, exercising and meditation are still very beneficial to this day. Since my latest surgery I am now back to regular exercise and feeling stronger everyday.

I feel the focus of replenishing in my chest, for more than one reason. The medical trauma I have endured has been on my chest and my rehabilitation is centered there. Also, the chest holds the heart and the chakras that hold love. For the longest time I felt very confused as to why I was chosen for the journey I am on. It made me resentful and questioning my faith that all things happen for a reason. I feel the work I am currently doing is replenishing to my core energy and where I have been physically compromised. I want to be an example to others who may walk this journey that you can overcome anything with humor and perseverance.

I have never thought of it in this way, but I definitely feel replenished at this stage of my healing. I have a new purpose and focus as to what I want this journey to mean. I don't think I have been put through all that I have gone through for no reason. I have always thought there must be a purpose for this suffering, and I am currently opening my energy to receive direction for that purpose."

With the stories of these two women you can see how easily the balance of our bodies can succumb over decades.

Activity and Tips:

This is where you use your emotions as a power source. Start with the declaration:

I am me! Then make a list of your achievements. Literally it can be anything that you've done.

- **I rode a bike for the first time in 30 years**
- **I didn't scream at my kids today**
- **I launched a new business**

Now how did ***that*** feel? Here is another great story of bearing the weight of others' burdens, releasing, empowering oneself and living in overflow.

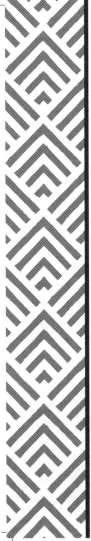

GUIDE TO CREATING BETTER HABITS

Begin with
Thank You!
List why you
are grateful

_____
_____
_____
_____
_____

THEN ASK YOURSELF AND JOURNAL ON THESE
QUESTIONS:
WHAT DO I DESIRE TO CREATE TODAY?

_____
_____
_____
_____

WHO DO I NEED TO BE TODAY?

_____
_____
_____
_____

WHAT DO I NEED TO ALIGN WITH TODAY?

_____
_____
_____
_____

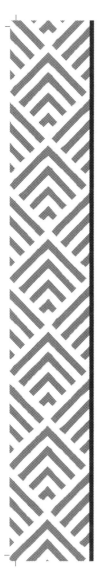

START WHERE YOU ARE

LIST

Pledge to
choose
better:
_____
_____
_____
_____
_____

HABITS THAT ARE SERVING ME WELL:

_____
_____
_____
_____

HABITS THAT ARE NOT SERVING ME:

_____
_____
_____
_____

HABITS WHICH ARE BETTER:

_____
_____
_____
_____

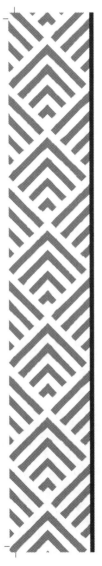

HOW CAN IT GET BETTER

L I S T

Pledge to
choose
better: _____
_____
_____
_____

HABITS WHICH ARE BETTER

_____
_____
_____

HABITS THAT ARE SERVING ME:

_____
_____
_____
_____

HABITS WHICH ARE BEST:(COMBINE THEM)

_____
_____
_____

CHAPTER 4

RESTRUCTURE: THE 5 STEPS TO SELF NURTURING

Quote:

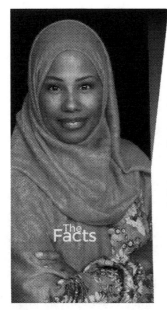

Imagine the best otherwise it's energy lost!

Loving the world when you are hurt is the best way to heal. There is so much joy and beauty to appreciate and hold in your heart that it squeezes out all of the pain.

~ Cordelia Gaffar

Main Idea: This is the step where you create sustainable self-nurturing habits to honor your body, mind and soul. By doing this important step, you will discover what your true personal values are.

Anecdote:

"I highly recommend signing up for the entire program, the benefits you will receive are priceless. I had an immeasurable amount of success with the Replenish Me ™ program and I will sign on again

> *because it was truly eye opening for me as a women's empowerment leader, learning how my mental, physical, emotional, spiritual beliefs, relationships, eating habits, etc..."*

Kisa struggled with her sleep before she started working with me. She would sleep a full 4-6 hours every night with fist clenched. Clenching the fist tightly in sleep is a sign of emotional anxiety and increased stress, can be related to a reaction to cholesterol medication and underlying medical conditions like rheumatoid arthritis. Rheumatoid arthritis is a condition middle aged women are often diagnosed with no known cause. However, according to Dr. Christaine Northrup is the accumulation of years of frustration from taking on other people's burdens. As a nurse by profession and divorced grandmother living with her single daughter she definitely nurtured everyone in her life more so than herself. The first step of Replenish Me ™ is to release what's expected and accepted by others in your life. This step took us almost four weeks and at the end of that time she immediately noticed that she stopped waking with clenched fists and felt well rested in the morning. Then she noticed that it was easier for her to eat breakfast in the morning and eased into regular daily exercise. Overall she was able to make choices that were self-nurturing focused and self-compassion based. As a result, she started speaking easily and freely for what she truly desired to happen in the moment. I saw her come alive and realize that she was time-rich. She had more time for her passion and side non-profit that she is building. Even within that space, she is now showing up more powerfully as a leader.

So what is different? Sleep is THE metabolic stabilizer. When she sleeps well, her mindset, food and movement choices support her energy. As a result she can also feels about herself, more confident and is more calm.

Here's what Kisa said and she also put it on my <u>LinkedIn</u> and <u>Facebook page</u>...

Information and application:

- Sleep
- Thoughts
- Food
- Exercise
- Emotions

Let's Talk About Your Immune System...Is it what you are eating? Your sleeping habits? Other habits? Or is it your thoughts? Journal over the next few days. Your immune system is based in our stomach. In fact, 90% of disease comes from digestive issues. When you don't sleep well or on time and enough it affects how you process the food we eat. The food you eat also plays a role in our energy levels which is directly related to oxygen production. You can always boost our oxygen with movement which is directly related to our circulation. However, here's the showstopper....your thoughts! Even if you eat well and exercise, the weight of your thoughts can throw off the whole show. How do you control that? Control is a strong word so how about you choose differently or better? So just for today, let's focus on sleep :)

Nurturing Tip #1 Sleep

We take it for granted and think that we only need sleep. As I discussed in the live session, sleep is a metabolic stabilizer whereas regular rest for each part of us is an overall system balance and there are also several types of rest we need to support our sleep. How much sleep is right for your body type? Contrary to popular belief everybody does not need 8 hours of sleep. The key is that the sleep be solid and uninterrupted. Let's first understand the sleep cycles. The first cycle of 90 minutes is your body calming. It is not abnormal to wake in the night but if it is abrupt and with a start then you may need a sleep time routine.

A great sleep time routine begins with breakfast. Front load your meals heavier meals meaning breakfast and lunch or at least lunch.

Eating less later in the day helps your body calm down and work less to prepare for the major overnight detox. Also limit refined sugar and caffeine after lunch and increase water intake. Also try to soak in a warm tub with lavender essential oil, epsom salt and Himalayan salt. It helps the detoxing and calming process to start.

Two hours before sleep, turn off all forms of screen (phone, reading devices, laptop and TV, etc. Only take warm water after and no more food from two hours before sleep.

Here are some more things to consider:

1. Everything you do in your day is cumulative
2. How much blue light exposure during the day and two hours before sleep
3. How much physical activity during the day
4. What are you eating?
5. How much stress in your day and what are you doing to deal with it?

How is your sleep now?

If you have problems falling to sleep, get curious as to why. Does the list below describe your sleep patterns and strategies for getting to sleep? If you truly struggle with sleep, would you call it insomnia (habitual sleeplessness; inability to sleep)? What causes insomnia?

- *Life events i.e. parties*
- *Furlows Interrupted*
- *Broken relationships*
- *Continuous stressful situations*
- *Current sleep/calm down routine*
- *Sleep aids*
- *Cannabis*
- *CBD oil*

- *Shower*
- *Writing down a daily schedule to remember*
- *Need creative rest*
- *Chronic fatigue resting in vertigo*

As long as this list is the cause is all hormonal imbalance. The solution is also quite simple:

Solutions:

Detoxify
Create a Calm Down Routine

I mentioned some elements of creating a sleep routine above and here are some more things to consider integrating below.

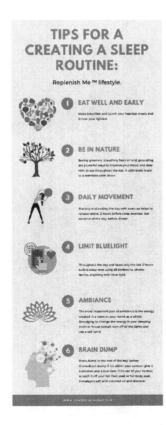

Tips for a Creating a Sleep Routine:

(I recommend to start only with the ones with * and build on it or use as needed.)

- 2 hours before sleep stop using all devices i.e. phone, laptop, anything with blue light*
- 2 hours before sleep exercise, last workout of the day, before dinner*
- Make breakfast and Lunch your heaviest meals and dinner your lightest*
- Brain dump at the end of the day, before dinner
- Brain dump if it's within your control, give it a solution and a due date. If it's out of your control, scratch it off your list.
- Journal at the end of the day but before dinner
- 1.5 before sleep eat last meal of the day*
- Listen to a podcast or meditation, do not lay down immediately after sleep
- Foot soak or full body soak, Himalayan salt with coconut oil and lavender
- Calcium Magnesium supplement*
- Water Chia seed water 4 oz. of warm water and ½ TBSP
- Grounding
- Smudging to change the energy in your sleeping room or house overall
- Turn off all the lights and use a salt lamp

If you wake in the middle of the night: (This is normal and how you are created as a human being so welcome it)

- Comfort yourself by praying or meditating
- Have a cup of herbal tea (comfrey, passion flower or skullcap)
- A calming activity like yoga or journaling

Keep a journal for your sleep journey

Nurturing Tip#2 - Let's Replenish and Boost Your Thoughts

THIS IS SIMPLE: Sweet talk ™ ...well it's really more than that!

To prepare for this step, start to journal your thoughts and notice how you are behaving. Notice your triggers and where you feel it in your body. Is it mostly your hips, neck, hands or back?

Yes, thinking is a full body activity. Did you know that most of our energy is sapped just by our thoughts? While you may have never noticed the correlation between your hip or knee pain with your thoughts, I will help to connect the dots and provide some techniques to release negative thoughts. Interestingly, it takes 5-7 positive thoughts to overcome one negative thought.

Pull out your journal and focus on:

- Thoughts and where you feel it in your body
- Connection between thoughts and the body
- Connection between conscious reframe with your words
- Create 5-7 positive thoughts to overcome each negative thought

How thoughts affect your immune system:

Let's talk about your thoughts and where you feel it in your body. What is the connection between thoughts and the body? Each energy center has a meaning. In the introductions, I showed you the chakras or energy centers and what they mean. Now I will give you context and a relatable meaning in your daily life. When you worry about what others think of you, it's literally a weight on your heart and back. For example, have you ever had an argument with your spouse, child or co-worker and found your thoughts weighing on you the rest of the day? There are two things happening there:

1. You have absorbed their negative energy
2. You are not allowing yourself to release your own.

I began this book with a story of extreme physical symptoms related to a heated exchange with a close friend, basically a completely toxic situation. Whilst my body was on alert in repair mode, my mind was ready with reinforcements in the "we know what to do mode". As I implemented the self-soothing massage, nourishing foods and sleep, I stopped my immune system from overreacting, my mind stopped racing and I was able to sleep and let it go. Some years ago, I found myself paralyzed emotionally desperately trying to resist grief over the loss of my father. During that time, my lungs were inflamed and I showed several symptoms of bronchitis. I was weak, achy, feverish and slept several hours. Dr. John Sarno, who I will discuss later in this book, sites cases of chronic pain where people have literally thought themselves into illness. In my weakened state, I went to the doctor who cleared me medically. Yes, I tested negative for bronchitis and was told to attend to my symptoms like the common cold. I had an epiphany just like after my OB had prescribed antidepressants for postpartum depression, I can cure myself with my nutrition, meditation, spiritual practices and movement. I decided to lean into it that I was able to overcome. I chose to lean into the love of my father and the wisdom he gave me. I reframed as I am with him in my wisdom not grief for his loss. Just by choosing to focus on thoughts of love over loss and fear, I was able to breathe easily again. I invite you also to reflect on what makes you truly happy - What did you do this week that truly made you happy? Capture the moment as it happens if possible.

We often hear that fear is not real or mind over matter. Of course, all of our feelings are real. What about mind in the matter? It is not in the denying of our feelings or situations it's in the being with them that brings forth the wisdom. In that connection with the body, we have a Body Soul Shift. The shift comes in creating a more powerful moment in your present to replace the negative one. In that process, you are effectively creating more than 5-7 positive thoughts to replace each negative one. In my grief example, I focused on the love and connection I had with my father. That helped me remember joyful moments and changed my physical state because I started to smile and laugh. In The

Power of Moments, Dan and Chip Health call it "moment-spotting". This habit is unnatural at some level because we just live and operate on autopilot. But when we start thinking in "moments", also known as being in the present, it allows us to slow down and recognize where the prose of life deserves celebrating. That's when we become the author of our own defining moments, start being in and with it thereby transforming it into a growth opportunity. As I often say, reframing our perspective with Sweet Talk ™. This gives us permission to use our emotions to build peak moments by:

> Boosting sensory appeal
> Fully experiencing our feelings like a child
> Change your vocabulary

The script you choose to express in words and actions how you feel the outward Sweet Talk ™ can create a whole new reality for you. Make today all about forgiveness. In your body, notice where you are holding on to your shoulds. Is it your shoulders? Neck? Or Lower Back? If it is your shoulders, that is the responsibility of others which you have chosen for yourself. Release it. If it is your neck, it is also related to taking on what is not yours but also ignoring what is. Be done with it If it is your lower back, it is old insecurities and struggles. Forgive it today start to see where you can be kinder to your body with forgiveness. It is the best way to release and be free.

Thoughts for the road:

- Pause and examine the thought
- Is it true? Is there space for self-compassion or self-forgiveness? Replace the thought with "moment-spotting" higher quality thought
- Create a poem that is your Sweet Talk ™ mantra to create your happy bubble

Nurturing Step #3 Let's Replenish and Boost With Food

Do you find yourself Stress eating? Find cooking overwhelming and end up at the fast food drive thru you swore off? Now are you feeling guilty that you succumbed again? Stop the madness!

- What are you eating?
- Does it support your immune system?
- How to make better choices to support your immune system?

"Eat like a Queen for breakfast, princess for lunch and lady's maid for dinner"~ modified by Cordelia

Better breakfast: If you don't eat breakfast, remember that you haven't eaten for several hours and you must break your fast. It's not about it being morning, it's about replenishing your body for all of the work it's been doing all night long. I get it! I've gone through periods when I could eat immediately after waking. Make sure that you start with plain warm water. That will get the body going and welcome the opportunity to consider food. Yes, it's like coaxing a teenager sometimes. Within the first half hour of waking have a good balance of good fats (coconut oil, nuts, seeds, boiled eggs, avocado), protein (cooked dark leafy greens, seeds, chia seeds) and carbs (bread won't kill you).

Better snacks: Reach for fruit, nuts and seeds. The combination of hydrating fruits, proteins and fats will do wonders for your energy levels.

Better breaks: Make sure to take a break at the end of every hour to do jumping jacks, walk around the block or some type of movement.

Nourishing without food: Let's talk about intermittent fasting. First of all if it's new to you for women, it's recommended to start every other day or try fasting one or two days per week. One more very important point about fasting as a woman is it's best not to do it during your menstrual cycle. During your menses, your body's working overtime to detoxify already so you will run it into the ground without a source of iron, calcium, magnesium, fats, carbohydrates, hydration and so many other essential minerals and vitamins. Scientifically, your iron stores are lower and dehydration is imminent. However, leading up to your cycle it may be a help in the regular detoxification process that comes with it. As a Muslim during my menstrual cycle, I neither pray or fast as this is a natural time of rest and deep connection to the mercy. I am mentioning this because I notice that I have more energy than usual when I fast prior to my cycle but you should test that theory. There is so much more I can say on this topic and it is a very integral part of the Replenish Me ™ process. Below I am providing a brief overview of how knowing your body type can help you truly understand how to create nutritional and lifestyle sustainable nurturing practices. As a Tibb Practitioner, we identify people by their humour or body type. Tibb means medicine and healing of the physical, mental and spiritual realms. Tibb physicians focus on harmonizing, assisting and encouraging and even love each person, each patient and guide him or her back to the condition of human happiness and wellness in the six lifestyle areas. The six lifestyle areas are air, food and drinks, physical activity, sleep and wakefulness, emotions and feelings and retention of fluids and evacuation of wastes. While what I study is based on the compilations of Avicenna, also known as Ibn Sina, who wrote 276 books including the Book of Impartial Judgment, The Book of Healing and the Canon of Medicine, this goes back to Hippocrates. Hippocrates is called the father of medicine and the namesake of the Hippocratic Oath. He relied on the body's own healing mechanisms rather than introducing external agents. His viewpoint is that disease is the occurrence of severe difficulty in digestion or pepsis of the environment of an organism. Ibn Sina developed this further by integrating the elements and season to more accurately identify body types. If you are interested in knowing more about your body type and how to use this method for your full benefit, I invite you to go to www.cordeliagaffar.com and to take the quiz on my site. I will follow up with a complimentary assessment report. The four humours are:

Phlegmatic - element is water and season winter.
Choleric - element is fire and season summer

Sanguine - element is air and season spring
Melancholic - element is earth and season autumn

In summary for this section on replenishing and boosting your immune system with food, be mindful to select foods that can support the immune system with every mouthful and replenish you with every meal. It is so important to start the day well and continue that for each meal as best possible. Also as we have discussed in the section on sleep, less food as the day goes on is better. Frontload all of your carbohydrates so that you are burning those sugars out before the body needs to calm down for the night.

Nurturing Step #4 Let's Replenish and Boost with Movement!

Do you exercise? If so, when? If not, why? You are doing great!

Let's dive into:

– Are you moving and how?
– Does your current level of activity support your immune system?
– How exercise supports your immune system?

Again this is one of the things to remember to power up with exercise its about:

Timing (before first meal, at least)
Quality- do it with great and intentional form
Consistency - must do it daily with weights every other day

This is the beginning of tapping into your inner wisdom. You're knowing that shows you how to take command of your life. One choice, one moment at a time, you step wisely into being more grateful. Everyday focus on the fact that you know what you need, how to get it, and how to solve it. This will help you in the face of negative opposition whether from inner chatter or external noise. When you inhale, inhale your knowing and exhale your confusion. Sometimes you need some help with the internal environment. Essential oils are an awesome way to do that. Peppermint helps with clarity. Sandalwood with grounding and lavender with calm...but take it easy with the lavender. In large quantities, it has also been known to stimulate. It doesn't have to be a special brand, just therapeutic grade. Try moving everyday. Track how you move daily.

If you are interested in knowing more about your body type and how to use this method for your full benefit, I invite you to go to www.cordeliagaffar.com and to take the quiz on my site. I will follow up with a complimentary assessment report.

Nurturing Step #5 Let's Replenish and Boost Your Emotions

Having gone through this process through the steps, do you feel replenished and stronger?

Journal how you have reframed your perspective. Look at how you react or choose not to in triggering situations. Are you choosing wholesomeness daily? Eating breakfast? Moving? Using essential oils to help? My hope is that you have had a major perspective shift and are on your way to a major breakthrough.

Notice:

- The connection between thoughts and emotions
- The connection between body and emotions
- See the connection between gratitude and emotions
- How it affects your immune system

Gratitude is something delicate and simple but truly powerful. It is at the root of all solutions. If you want to reduce stress, eat better, be more productive, or even release weight, it all starts with a grateful heart. A grateful heart starts with a positive mindset.

Self - Compassion, movement, being grounded, in the moment, pauses, understanding how to listen to when you need what foods, when you need which types of movement or rest so you can maintain your energy throughout the day. The work of Dr. John Sarno has a 75-85% success rate in healing back and neck pain and fibromyalgia related to TMS or tension myositis syndrome. "He notes that the personalities of those who tend to get this syndrome are characterized by being highly conscientious, responsible, and perfectionistic. "What he has found is that our pain is associated with not being able to "stomach" certain emotions and disowning parts of our bodies for one reason or another. In this program you will learn how to literally speak to your body and pain and release it. When we think of how we are structured physiologically, we can see that if one system is off it affects the rest. According to Miranda Esmonde White, "a state of well-being is the absence of illness, injury, pain, chronic exhaustion, and mental depression. Good health or well-being would also include plenty of energy to carry us throughout our busy days, and help us maintain a positive outlook. Perfection is a myth. It's about implementing self-nurturing practices which create a habit of consciousness to the alert systems of the body and recognizing and eventually becoming proactive in knowing the seasons for each. Write where you felt resistance in your body the most. Ever wonder how to get away from the chaotic inner chatter and to truly step into your purpose in this world? It's like no matter how hard you try and no matter what you do, you are just stuck! Sometimes you just need something to move you...something that you already possess...something hiding...It is your inner wisdom! We all have it but suppress it when we do not take time for gratitude. You may be thinking, "that's a leap! "It is not. Most very successful people have a practice of meditating on having a grateful heart. Try it when you walk with an attitude of gratitude: get you unstuck quiet that inner negative chatter creates a firm boundary for external negativity and most of all...awakens your inner wisdom.

In summary, a grateful heart starts with a positive mindset the day. My signature program, Replenish Me ™ is built on its foundation. This past week is only a drop in the ocean of the possibilities, you can achieve with the full course. Connect to your body to check in with where you feel resistance or pain. Notice the affected energy center and think of the story associated with that body part. Be grateful for that lesson and accept you as you are. Reframe your thoughts surrounding negative experiences and rewrite with the exact opposite. By reframing your perspective with gratitude you are helping your body to heal and your immune system to be stronger. Continue to journal your journey. Capture what you are grateful for, struggling with, ways to choose positive words surrounding triggering life events, old stories, and understand that people project their stories on you and you don't have to accept it. In fact, your shoulders will feel lighter if you don't! If you are interested in knowing more about your body type and how to use this method for your full benefit, I invite you to go to www.cordeliagaffar.com and to take the quiz on my site. I will follow up with a complimentary assessment report.

Now that you have all the tools you need to Replenish and Boost Your Immune System through achieving better sleep, thoughts, food, movement and emotions, use this book as an ongoing resource. Replenish Me ™ steps:

- — Release
- — Restructure
- — Refresh
- — Rebirth

Expertise:

The key to your spiritual, emotional and physical health is through sustainable self-nurturing practices. Replenish Me ™ is the process to unlearn behaviors which are keeping you stressed out and in a cycle of self-neglect. Through Replenish Me ™ you can become who you are meant to be! The world needs you to stop rolling over and to start standing up for yourself. It's time to stop negotiating against yourself. When you meet your needs, you can show up powerfully!

This chapter the activities were included above.

CHAPTER 5

HOW YOUR BODY TELLS YOU TO REFRESH YOUR RELATIONSHIPS

Quote:

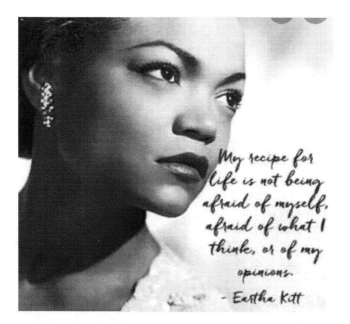

My recipe for life is not being afraid of myself, afraid of what I think, or of my opinions.

- Eartha Kitt

Main Idea: In this chapter, I'm sharing personal stories in my life of how I knew that I needed to refresh my intimate relationship and the significance of the signs in my body and minor behavioral changes. As you read my story, see yourself.

Anecdote:

During the time I was writing this book, life was less than kind. I posted this on Facebook:

"It's been a rough month for me because when I'm not inspiring the world I'm a wife and a mother. Even after 21 years of marriage we have some knock down drag outs, literally.

So I have the opportunity of using my emotions as a power source daily. Without self-compassion, self-forgiveness and self-belief, I would crumble and die with a shattered heart. All that glitters isn't gold. Disentangling isn't easy or a streamlined process. It's practicing love in all forms of detachment while healing all while empowering and inspiring your children to have emotional mastery. Some of what I'm saying may be triggering for those of you who understand and confusing for those of you who don't get it or default to judgment. Either way I'm sharing this message for those of you who need it. I have moments when I completely want to give up and cave into the defeat and negative suggestions. But living in this world as an intuitive and highly sensitive person only has made me stronger and able to see through the fog of the matrix of narcissists, haters and blockers. So I rise after pouring back into myself with love, trust, high quality nutrition, nature walks, and cuddles with my children.

What do you do when it gets to be too much?"

The responses were mostly opening that conversation about healthy ways to deal with life. However, there were three who wanted to "help" me. They recommended that I cower to my husband's shallow ego for the benefit of the healing of the children. In that same conversation I was called," conniving, defiant and manipulative". I was told that I must "preserve" the family. I was instructed to come up with a plan that didn't include assuming that my business would flourish. NO matter what anyone said I knew in my mind and body that it was time to do something drastic and very different! There were so many signs. The mindless way I would do things that I normally would be very intentional with like eating. The result of mindless eating yielded a sign. For example, when I went to Dallas, I had an awesome dinner with a friend and enjoyed my meal so much that I bit my fork with the food on it all while trying to speak....What does that equal? A chipped tooth! Well at least that's what I saw. However, when I went to my dentist the next week, I found out that I have hairline fractures on three of my teeth. She said even though my teeth are otherwise healthy, it's better to correct them. Wow! It made me think about how sometimes you don't see the little cracks in your life. Although you experience things that challenge your values, you overlook it or blatantly ignore it. When you don't pause with each infraction, you may acknowledge several "lesser struggles", like a chipped tooth, yet choose to judge yourself rather than to see yourself. In the end, you wonder why that little thing breaks you. When in fact what really happened was that over time you become more and more uncomfortable and again ignore or choose to numb it until it becomes unbearable.

Here's one last and more explicit example of what I was explaining. On a hike, I had to navigate very slippery muddy rocks. I was at the top of a 60 foot drop. I was literally forced to stay in each moment to step carefully. I viewed it from the growth perspective of "stay in the present and don't worry too much about what's coming up, if you can do this you can do that". I finally realized that this has been my pattern of swinging between stagnation or fixed mindset and transformation or growth mindset. This is why I love hiking! It is mental practice for literally moving better through life. I realized in my life that I give away my power in the form of being in life situations that keep my eyes so focused on the now in a fearful way. As in if I don't figure out how not to fall in the spot where I'm standing I could suffer greatly or die. When I could also view the same situation as a learning opportunity. I allowed myself to get caught up in my mind only to hold on to that which is fleeting...this body. The whirlwind that becomes a barrier to self-compassion is the fear of losing or not having possessions or human relationships. So I free fall into abundance and allow myself to be grateful for gravity which will not allow me to fall and die neither during my hike nor in my life. Collectively these experiences awakened me to see that it was time to refresh my most intimate relationship.

Information:

Breathe into that! Be with your emotions, be free!

Self-compassion is more than a catch phrase it's life. Being raised with love and compassion created a bubble for me and is my safety net when my life seems scary or impossible. Love really can overcome fear, anger, hate and so much more. I'm a testament to that. That's why I know that when we lean into our darkest and most difficult emotions, especially as women, we are so much more powerful!

Compassion literally means: sympathetic pity and concern for the sufferings or misfortunes of others and comes from Latin *compassio(n-)*, from *compati* 'suffer with. Suffer with the darkness you experience in life and have sympathy for yourself. That is the path to freedom rather than to numb, avoid or ignore them. In the last chapter, I introduced the work of Dr. John Sarno, who originated the term tension myositis syndrome (TMS) to name a psychosomatic condition producing pain, particularly back pain. 99% of the women I work with complain of some form of back pain. My focus for superficial prognosis is identifying the affected energy center associated with your pain or the place where your body responds most frequently to adversity. What he has found is that our pain is associated with not being able to "stomach" certain emotions and disowning parts of our bodies for one reason or another. Literally that means just by your thoughts you believe "ill" of certain parts and they suffer the neglect of your resulting actions. Dr. John Sarno has healed thousands of patients of chronic back pain by helping them acknowledge the repressed rage in their unconscious. It's the shadow work process.

Yes your words are creating a physical reality. It also works the other way round as in creating energy in your body to create a sense of well-being. Essentrics ™ is the modality I've used for over 15 years which focuses on activating your mitochondria, the powerhouse of our cells. When we think of how we are structured physiologically, we can see that if one system is off it affects the rest. According to Miranda Esmonde White, the creator of Essentrics ™, "a state of well-being is the absence of illness, injury, pain, chronic exhaustion, and mental depression. Good health or well-being would also include plenty of energy to carry us throughout our busy days, and help us maintain a positive outlook." When I say lean into your emotions as a power source, I literally mean that! Your emotions are chemical reactions in the body which last up to 90 seconds. In the brief period of time, thoughts fill your mind associated with the feelings in your cells. You have a choice to react to each negative thought or to notice the chemical reaction, focus on that and physically brace yourself. I tell my clients if you are standing, strike a Wonder Woman pose. If you are sitting, sit up straight and hold onto a table or your desk. Then breathe. Allow the thoughts, if any to come through. If they are overwhelmingly negative and hang out select only one and cross examine it. That inner dialogue goes like this:

Negative thought, "Oh shit! This is really bad! It's going to cause…"

Conscious cross examination," In this moment what is actually happening?"

Negative thought," Nothing, but it will!"

Conscious cross examination," In this moment everything is peaceful. At this moment you have choices. You can choose differently"

This is Sweet Talk ™. This is the refresh step.

Application:

What comes up for you? Where do you feel it in your body? Do you feel it in your body?

Over the years, I've gotten a variety of responses as you can imagine.

"Emotions make you weak!"

"I feel nothing anywhere in my body"

"I feel it in my hips"

All these responses tell me volumes about who I'm talking to. Before I reveal their true identities, let me give you some background. We have been institutionalized, I know that's a strong word, to believe that there is a time and place for emotions. There are parameters of expression as well determined by your age, gender, and other categories. However, what my clients have proven to me is that when you let go of what is accepted and expected you are more courageous therefore more powerful. One woman I worked with always wanted to "keep the peace" and serve her patients at the high level. So she would linger and listen to their complaints to the point of physical and emotional overwhelm. Once she even allowed one patient to begin a tirade and she started to have a tingling in her shoulders and a tightening in her heart. A sign she knows means that she was starting to deeply connect to their story in a way that takes her focus off of her expertise and wears her out physically. At home, she would repeat the same pattern not speaking up for her need to be poured back into. Again she felt the abandonment of no one feeling her exhaustion and frustration with having to continue to serve at home. This started in the lower back and right then left knee pain. By extension in her community service efforts, again she was an emotional martyr. Her explanation to herself was, "I am supposed to do these things and not expect anything in return". This caused a full system shutdown in a way that she couldn't sleep well at night. She feels it everywhere in her body because the way emotions work is they are actual peptide chains which exist in every cell of our body. As someone who cares deeply for people, she connects to people and prioritizes their emotions over hers. That causes the emotional overwhelm. She could easily honor her heart by stopping the person as she begins to feel the tingling in her shoulders, she has a choice to say" I completely feel how uncomfortable you are right now. Let me make a plan to sort you."

More than likely she is familiar with their story and has the expertise to support without hearing too much detail. If this sounds like you, it's time to refresh and make new choices. After working with me using the Replenish Me ™ process she had peaceful sleep and used her voice to speak up for what honors her.

Another woman, who was a powerful corporate executive, would endure having her brilliant ideas either batted down by her superiors and peers or overlooked only for them to later resurface as the contribution of a male counterpart or even worse the CEO himself. She feared speaking up because she was so overwhelmed with anger she couldn't "intelligently articulate at an educated level". At the slightest tremor of her hand, she rushes off to the gym to work it out of her system. She is telling herself, 'Successful women stay the course and don't whine'. Although when her male peers spoke out of turn and with full on rage, their ideas and recognition were realized. She then maps out a new plan of attack and suppresses her anger with a glass of wine, just one not to affect her waistline. When I asked her where she feels it in her body, she said not at all. Whilst we applaud her "showing up as a strong" woman, she is an example of classic freeze and that weakens the mind and body over time.

During the COVID 19 lockdown, I have a client who is feeling out of step because she loves the control of certainty. Now she is not in control of her time, because the husband and children are home, and is in constant worry for her health and that of her family. She is in a state of complete anxiety. For her it always started in her lower back or stomach. But she would self medicate by staying up late binge eating or 'comfort food exploring 'as she called it. She closely represents flight.

Which one are you? What does it all mean?

When you are on freeze, it means that you are less inclined to tolerate uncertainty and constantly desire control and certainty. Decades of research on the etiology of worrying have suggested that uncertainty intolerance is actually the root cause of worry and generalized anxiety disorder. This is because the person who accepts uncertainty acknowledges that they are not in absolute control of their affairs and does not stress over what they cannot control. Conversely, the one who runs away from uncertainty and covets control over the details of their life will find "what they resist to persist." They will find uncertainty everywhere and be in a perpetual state of worry, anxiety, and stress. Stress is a direct response to situations where people feel uncertain and feel a lack of control. Worrying and anxiety then lead to fear, and fear leads people to overestimate the risk of negative outcomes. This creates a negative feedback cycle that perpetuates anxiety. Thus, not only does uncertainty intolerance cause us to worry about today, through increased anxiety and fear we envision a future far more dismal than it actually will be. This creates a sense of hopelessness and pessimism about the future.

For example, three different outlooks regarding effects of the coronavirus:

1. Seeing the potential of blessings resulting from its spread;
2. Expressing concern for oneself, others, and society;
3. Pessimistically predicting that, over the next few months, things will unfold largely negatively.

Higher uncertainty intolerance the lower your mental health. Perception acts as a lens through which we view reality, and it influences what we focus on, our interpretation of life events, and the decisions we subsequently make. This is a perfect place to apply Sweet Talk ™, the vocabulary and words that honor the value of your very essence and all of those possibilities over the common world view, opinion of others or perceived reality. Opportunities to reimagine the world and one's place within it. Write down your biggest failure and what you learned from it. Kind of like life we can appear to be on top which is lonely but when we see the humanity in each other we truly win. That's why I say women are the pillars of society and our power is leaning into our emotions. This situation is the perfect opportunity to turn your habit of emotional numbing and avoiding to embracing. That's the only way to truly have courage and be strong for humanity. When was the last time you took the time to be with your feelings?

Activity:

Allow the fall of emotions to envelope your body. Have you let your blood pulse and pump into your thighs and knees and toes? You know when it's not just your face that feels hot?

Self is the most powerful force to develop and we have an entire lifetime to do it. When we honor our spiritual connection, it is the highest form of expressing self-nurturing. We are spirits having a human experience. The part of us which connects to this world is the mind. That is where our soul and emotions live. It's that limbo land between body and mind. Self-compassion is loving what honors you so much that only love comes to you And that's why when we focus on love in its purest form, we find that it is pure detachment.

Self-belief is as your true self because that's the Best You and detaching from other's opinions

Self-worth is valuing you without a measuring scale

Self-forgiveness is giving yourself grace for growing, evolving and blossoming and leaning into that which honors you

Self-trust is showing for yourself no matter what in full capacity

Free yourself and be yourself with deep "love", which my sweet talk and be detached. Receiving and gratitude become a flow instead of a dam blocked by our self-doubt or desperation. Transformation begins with you. See yourself as you desire to be and keep your vision fixed on that. Everything you desire will flow to you in that vibration. Do you see yourself in my story? Reflect as you make choices.

CHAPTER 6

REFRESH: DECODING DETACHMENT

Quote:

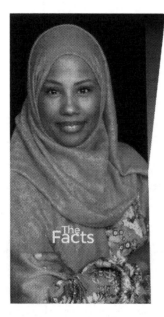

"Whenever we manage to love without expectations, calculations, negotiations, we are indeed in heaven."

-Rumi

Main Idea: How do you detach while being love?

Anecdote:

Marriage is the ultimate relationship to use as a way to refresh who is honoring your values and deserves to be in your inner circle. Sometimes for years, you go with the status quo and remain in a miserable, toxic or even abusive relationships for decades. I really thought divorce meant failure. My parents never divorced and were happy. Yet if this marriage were to end, it would be my second time and I struggled with what that meant for me on a worthiness level. Having spent most of our marriage heavily engaged in self-development on a spiritual, emotional and physical level, I knew it was time to re-write that story and create a new muscle memory. We created and raised six children together. Over the years, I connected more deeply with the Divine and focused on Allah as the source of my joy and pleasure. As the years passed I better understood how to activate my own pleasure centers and expected more of a spiritual high over a physical one. I chose when I would conceive. The spacing went from every two years to three and then four years with our last child. Even before I was certain that our marriage would end, I desired the disentanglement to be one of grace and dignity.

I'm the type of person who needs to see signs preferably in nature of how it will definitely sort. In a perfect world, I would love my beloved to communicate openly and clearly. However, the innuendos from nature played a double *entendre* in the final days and even immediately afterwards. For me the days afterwards thrust me into a disentangling project. At the beginning of the summer, my husband had the grand idea of planting a garden with peppers, tomatoes, cucumbers and broccoli. However, like our life together everything entangled and over grew even while dead and diseased things were being held onto in the mix. In the early stages it was mostly directing the small vines with short sticks. However, somewhere between the heavy rains and the heavy whirlwinds that brought our life together to a halt, the tomatoes had gotten taller than their binds, the broccoli struggled for light and the cucumbers flourished underneath it all.

The week after he moved out, as best I could I rerouted the tomato plants into the cages so that they have a chance at life. We have been able to enjoy cucumbers through all the fray. Interestingly, cucumbers like the under rumblings of our unraveling marriage create vines to keep themselves entangled with the tomatoes and actually fuse. The symbolism was so very uncanny for me. I was determined to break the cucumbers free of their chosen path killing neither the tomatoes nor themselves. However, the tomatoes were too strong to die even though the cucumbers wouldn't allow them to stand and grow or have enough light to turn red. The cucumbers relied on the cover of its own leaves and those of the tomato plants. In the end, I am represented in the tomato plants in my garden and the final three years of our life together was exactly like my rerouting the tomatoes with care and love and detachment.

Expertise

"Love is multidimensional
It's the is lift in your chest as you breathe
The pause in your day even when its been less than sensational
It's the choice you make with each hello
The gift of elevation and presence rendering you inspirational
It's can be YES and mostly your NO"

~Cordelia Attwell Gaffar

Information: Self-Actualization is Really Detachment

We are familiar with this model of the hierarchy of where the human being aspires to reach. This is more of a westernization of Eastern concepts that are intangible. Once all of basic needs are met, we seek love and belonging. For women, this piece is a double edged sword. We seek it from our significant other and from peers. Although, we tend to feel judged by other women and rarely have a sense of belonging. Even in my circles sometimes we hide our love for one another rather than loving unconditionally.

In turn that affects our esteem. It causes us to peak here and linger, continuously reinventing ourselves to fit the mold of others to perhaps belong or be accepted. Instead this is where we should detach from the concept of belonging and love ourselves unconditionally. Thereby making loving and belonging to others seamless.

If we can achieve that, will that mean that we have self-actualized?

I believe not. As I started with, self-actualization is really detachment. It is true love. It is tied to evolving and connecting to our spiritual selves. Knowing our soul, shifting our bodies into that and having the self-confidence to just be no matter what. At the top is the Sweet Talk ™.

That is the bubbling up of your genuine soul and spiritual being. The embracing of the spiritual self in the physical world. This is how we retrain or refresh our inner circle. In order to make space for new habits we must get rid of the old. That requires true reprogramming and detachment. To support you, I have taken the word DETACHMENT and created an acronym. I invite you to dedicate a week to feeling into each word. At the end of the chapter I will give you an exercise to implement.

D is for Detachment

Once upon a time, I cared so much about my job that I would soften my boundaries to be there even though I had an eight week old baby. When I had discussed my maternity leave, back in 2000, we had agreed that I could work from home. Those were the days of dial up and the complaint from the top was that my reports were constantly delayed. At that time, I was a Senior Accountant for a new IT startup. So in theory they had access to correct the situation.

As a new mom, I ramped up on juggling nursing, diapering, eating and being available for call pretty quickly and imagining in the dial-up world! As a new wife, I even worked in cooking and laundry and cleaning in the mix.

In those days, I was so attached to approval with my boss and my husband that when either expressed disapproval, I was resentful to say the least. I continued to "prove" myself and spin in circles until I was laid off. Then I was devastated! My thoughts spiraled with:

'How could they...when I was working so hard...?

Don't they know that, I ignored my daughter's cries sometimes

I burned the dinner which caused arguments with my husband

And this...!'

Do you ever feel like no one appreciates anything you do? Especially when you feel that you are giving it your all? It's difficult enough to have all of these plates spinning but to not even be acknowledged!??

What the gift of being laid off brought was detachment.

I decided if I were to work again, and I took my sweet time with my job search, that I would do so on my terms. If they asked for anything outside of my job description or career path, I would stand my ground and not do it.

In the meantime, I connected to my daughter in a way that I learned to love unconditionally. We had a relationship without approval, disappointment or expectation. We were in sync. I knew by her movement and breath when she needed a diaper change or to eat or to be held or to play. It even got to the point that I stopped using diapers and put her over the sink because she was too small to sit on the toilet.

When I finally went back to work, I surprisingly got the job I desired pretty quickly because in the interview I wasn't attached to the outcome. If I was delayed with the daycare, I called ahead with "I'll be there in time to present at the meeting".

I'm sharing this story so that you see the power of detachment. It helps you to focus on your desires and what nourishes you. As I write this, I'm realizing that I've always been about the Replenish Me Reset.

The period between me losing one job and starting my new one was a very intensive four weeks, much like my Replenish Me Reset Program. In this time, I released the expectations of others, restructured my mindset, refreshed how I allowed people to treat me and rebirthed as a new woman.

E is for Ego

Are you feeling a pull against your heart for fear of rejection? Do you find yourself predicting the thoughts or misinterpretations of your friends and family when you go after what your heart truly desires?

That's your ego.

For thirteen years, my ego kept me silent and miserable. I was locked, trapped, muzzled and in the back of a closet. It was so severe that when I started to emerge, daylight hurt my eyes and the warmth of the sun sent me into retreat. Now, I will repeat that in English...I poked my head by writing my first book but hid by only doing workshops in familiar communities to sell it. Yes, I was doing a great service to my community and practicing proof of concept but if I am truly honest with myself I was not unlocking my true potential.

Transformation begins with you. See yourself as you desire to be and keep your vision fixed on that. Everything you desire will flow to you in that vibration.

So move your hips knowing that everyone is looking so make it count. Your ego will whisper, "you slut!...stop that!...what will they think?" Your body will feel free and your heart will beat with passion that you have forgotten.

Just yell back to ego, "I forgive you for not winding up more often publicly"...throw your head back and swirl in circles.

T is for Tether

What is your tether? What keeps you in this current place or situation and away from where you desire to be?

Feel into that thought for a moment and truly reflect.

Although, I passionately feel it has less to do with intellect.

It's all in your feelings that you may not detect.

It's all in your body, you're hard wired to respect social norms.

Tell me, what would it take to break those shackles that keep you in place.

Do you fear that you might go into outer space?

And if you did, yes it mightn't be commonplace,

But oh what adventures you'd have and at a crazy pace!

A is for Ascend

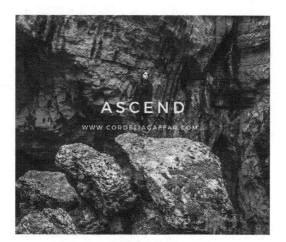

People are heavy with opinions and advice for ways to live your life. They'll tell you to sell your house, which car to buy and which clothes to wear all with your money. They'll tell you how to raise your kids, your dog and how to care for your ailing parents. In fact if we listened to the advice of others and actually valued it above our own opinions, values, and expertise on our own life, you might find yourself staying in a marriage you hate, closing a business you love and believe in and destroying your relationships with your children.

The great news is that you can rise above the noise.

You have a choice to believe that you are the expert of your life.

You have the power to Ascend!

No matter what anyone says and thinks, continue to climb higher.

C is for Curious

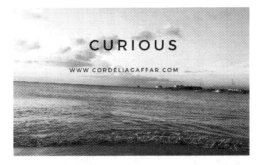

If you had ten minutes left to live how would you positively impact the world?

Or would you just give up and say, "it only ten minutes?

Would you spend impactful time with your children in hopes of influencing the next generation?

Would you change the way you express love with your partner, to shift his perspective of your relationship?

Would you simply have a sense of Curiosity fused with play and keep the secret to yourself? All the while exploring what you are capable of?

Or would you stare at the ceiling in regret of all the time you wasted?

Curiosity is such a beautiful thing

I see my younger children always at play, exploring new ways to challenge and entertain themselves and share that with each other. Watching then is my inspiration and motivation to think outside of the box and detach from what's expected.

So if I had ten minutes to live I'd be curious to see how I would choose to positively impact the world and encourage you to explore that everyday.

It's all about looking for the possibilities in a given situation and discovering how far you can exceed your limits.

H is for Heal

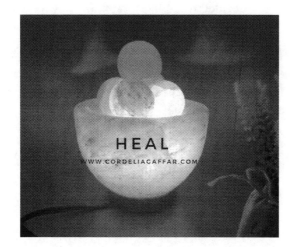

During the time that I am writing this book, I introduced Paul Laurence Dunbar's poem "We Wear the Mask " to my older children. It made me think about the process of healing. We can only begin to heal when we choose to stop wearing the mask. This poem is timeless and can be for any people although we know that Paul Laurence Dunbar was a renowned Black poet who wrote during the turn of the 20th century. He had to work as a janitor because Blacks during his time were not seen as articulate or intelligent.

As a woman, you may have experienced something similar. Or perhaps, you feel that you are considered less because you are an immigrant. Do you struggle with being your true self due to others perception? Are you so wrapped up in proving them wrong that you still show up as someone else? Are you triggered when you are with someone who may remind you of your less evolved self?

Consider this....Maybe you need to heal. Being worried about what people think needs to end and will not allow you to truly mend. Being insecure about stepping out and speaking your truth means you are still wearing a mask. What is it protecting you from? Is it truly protecting you? Recently, I had a stye for over two months for the first time in my life. Usually they disappear within a day or two. How could I do my Facebook lives? Record my podcast for my YouTube channel? After a few days, I decided to do live videos anyway. Eventually, I even started attending networking events without makeup. I literally became comfortable in my own skin as a result. This was an opportunity to truly embrace myself and reflect on my self perception.

What are you going through that has been an opening? Are you allowing it to be an opening?

If not, I invite you to try to heal.

M is for Mitochondria

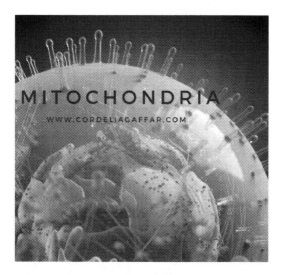

Mitochondria are the powerhouses for the essential cells in our bodies.[1] The way they work in the body is to generate power by converting energy into forms that are usable by that specific cell. In the fluid part of our cells, the mitochondria creates fuel from the foods we eat to help our bodies grow and detoxify. Structurally they are oblong and have a double membrane. Mitochondria are found in abundance in muscle, fat, and liver cells to provide the energy required for specific and vital activities. [2]This is a very important point to understand because these are the places in the body which take the brunt of our emotional trauma. That matters because they also have their own DNA and create their own proteins however unlike regular DNA is not self-repairing.

When I was mapping out the acronym for D.E.T.A.C.H.M.E.N.T., I wanted to be very specific about the meaning of the word as a whole and metaphorically. Therefore, when it came to M, I had to choose just the right word. I could have easily chosen muscle memory but emotions

---

[1] https://www.medicinenet.com/mitochondrial_disease/article.htm#what_is_the_prognosis_for_mitochondrial_disease

[2] https://www.thoughtco.com/mitochondria-defined-373367

are so much deeper than we currently comprehend. That's why I chose the word mitochondria and the many biology lessons.

So what does that mean?

When you experience unresolved emotional issues for an extended period of time, it depletes the mitochondrias abilities to get the fuel from your food to give each muscle (think movement and energy), liver (think detoxification system shut down), fat (think excessive storage) cell the power to function normally. That causes irreparable damage. The process of decline begins before the age of 20 and by the time it's noticeable severe decline is already happening. It appears with blood pressure and cardiovascular issues and lethargy in exercise routines and can lead to dementia and death.

Let me include a disclaimer here that I'm not recommending you are headed for dementia, high blood pressure or any other severe disease. However, I am inviting you to pay attention to your choices and behavior patterns when it comes to taking care of yourself. Is it possible that on a cellular level you are actually powering down?

So think again when you say that you don't want to exercise or don't have the energy to exercise. What is the deeper meaning? Although the choice may seem unconscious like "I don't feel like it today". I invite you to think again and be both conscious and honest with that choice.

Ask the curious questions:

Have you had an emotionally draining week? Day?

What is your pattern surrounding your decision to not exercise or not do something good for your body?

These are all rhetorical questions however, if you are inspired to please comment below or send me an email with your reflections.

My most profound response on *FB was by Tara Opie* "After reading, I better understand the importance of how holding on to unresolved issues can exacerbate health issues. My mother's family has a history of high blood pressure, dementia and vision issues. We have all learned to hold onto resentments and stress, emotional eating and fluctuating weight. Paired with, when considering self first, it could be viewed as selfish, making themselves martyrs can prove to be developed as procrastination and can lead to exhaustion."

And on *LinkedIn my Ike IkoKwo, CPA*" It's important to understand how negative emotions impact our physiology. Trauma is real and is stored in our brain, heart and GI tract. Getting to the question behind the question and understanding the meaning we give to every interaction we have in life is essential to understanding that we really create every experience and more importantly the meanings we attach to those experiences and how those meanings either haunt us and keep us bound or empower us and propel us to new heights of achievement. Great <u>article Cordelia</u>!³"

E is for Eliminate Transformation is about how to permanently #eliminate habits, choices, environments and relationships that are not serving you

N is for Nurture As you continue on our path to better love yourself, you may notice that you coddle and pay more attention to your intricacies and idiosyncrasies. Previously you may have shamed or harshly judged yourself for them whereas now you find them cute or alluring. You may sometimes even find yourself giggling for no reason.

Yes, giggling is a form of nurturing yourself. Do you remember being a young child? Remember when your mom and you made silly faces giggled? That's what you are now doing with yourself, for yourself and by yourself.

---

³ <u>https://www.linkedin.com/pulse/when-you-too-tired-exercise-cordelia-gaffar/?tra</u> <u>ckingId=x8KrV8GPv2GyY8HQL0MDpg%3D%3D</u>

By extension, the people in your close circle who don't mirror your new found self-compassion may naturally fade away or you desire less time with them. You are now standing up for the things that you were always too shy to mention or feared judgement from others.

Your inner chatter and outer vocabulary now match. No more wearing a mask or walking on eggshells. You are a woman of a certain age with a certain knowing.

Do you resonate with this? Which part do you wish you had more of?

T is for Transcend Abu Hurayra reported that the Prophet, may Allah bless him and grant him peace, said, "Wealth is not from a lot of money. Wealth is the independence of the self." [Agreed upon]

When you have completely detached from the material, you are independent. You are free to show up as your true self. The self you have been withholding from the world.

Application: Your turn to practice detachment.

Where in your life do you desire detachment? What patterns keep you entangled in your relationship or job? Connect to the source of pleasure and joy of the relationship or your job. Yes that's the Divine.

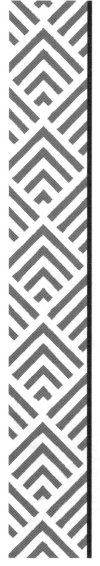

GUIDE TO REFRESH

Begin with what truly honors you

_____
_____
_____
_____
_____

LIFE SHRINKS OR EXPANDS ACCORDING TO ONE'S COURAGE~ ANAIS NIN

I COMMIT TO HAVING THE COURAGE TO HONOR ME

_____

_____

_____

_____

WHO SUPPORTS ME IN HONORING ME?

_____

_____

_____

_____

WHO DOES NOT SUPPORT ME IN HONORING ME?

_____

_____

_____

_____

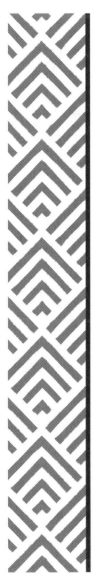

KEEP MY POWER

LIST

Pledge to
choose
better:

HOW HAVE I BEEN GIVING AWAY MY POWER?

HOW HAVE I BEEN STANDING IN MY POWER?

I COMMIT TO:

CHAPTER 7

BEGINNING TO REBIRTH

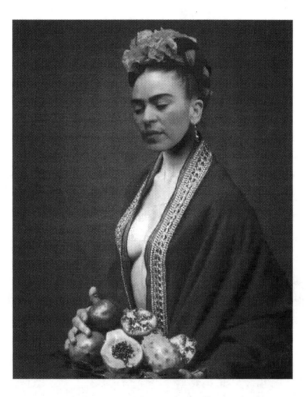

Quote: Frida Kahlo told her husband, "I'm not asking you to kiss me, nor apologize to me when I think you're wrong. I won't even ask you to hug me when I need it most. I don't ask you to tell me how beautiful I am, even if it's a lie, nor write me anything beautiful. I won't even ask you to call me to tell me how your day went, nor tell me you miss me. I won't ask you to thank me for everything I do for you, nor to care about me when my soul is down, and of course, I won't ask you to support me in my decisions. I won't even ask you to listen to me when I have a thousand stories to tell you. I won't ask you to do anything, not even be by my side forever. Because if I have to ask you, I don't want it anymore."

Main Idea: Choose your rebirth and strengthen those muscles even when it's hard.

Anecdote:

Just like that 24 hours later my midsection protruded accompanied by all of the angst and fear and trembling of trauma. Imagine just a simple argument gone awry and exploding into a severe disagreement. In the moment I seemed calm, cool and collected but that was just shock management at its best. In reality, I was on freeze as I had been for most of my marriage. Now I was free to freak out and grieve. Why can't I just sleep and can we just move on?

The next day I had to deal with my younger children being cranky and out of sync. Instead of a proper, reconciliation my husband and I proceeded as if nothing had happened. On his part, he did everything from making jokes in the car when we picked him up to finally doing things I had requested months before. He was lovable again and I felt ashamed of being angry at all. That was our dysfunctional way to resolve explosive situations. Silently, I was still connecting the triggers to outcomes. Then in the name of emotional wellness and overall self-nurturing, I left it. The reality of the situation was that I truly desired a world without anxiety attacks, clear skin, normal bowel function and peaceful nights. Ultimately I chose to soothe my nerves with a late night oatmeal, coconut oil and walnuts, it clutches my rib cage tight and unhinges my right side. That meant drinking warm water and learning to center and master my mindset. For me to exist and flourish without losing myself, I have earned to love and all things physical with detachment. Allowing myself to receive THE LOVE from the Source, Allah, so that there is an overflow. That overflow is for you to love yourself, walk in your purpose and be an example for your children. That was the gift of my marriage. I developed Sweet Talk ™ and the Happy Bubble Meditation ™. During my marriage these were coping mechanisms, but when I started my business they became tools. By using these two very powerful tools in my life, I radiated the detached love and pulled in what would not only free me from my marriage but my ultimate rebirth.

Information:

Our bodies cry in so many ways. Sometimes it's due to years of giving away our power through having sex with people who are not worthy of us. We have painful cramps, fibroids, cervical cancer. Sometimes through chronic STD which leads to cervical cancer. On top of the deep feeling of unworthiness that we borrow from those people we allow in our bodies, we are embarrassed to get the help we need to treat our physical expression of unworthiness and suffer physically, mentally, and emotionally until it actually kills us. Or maybe it's our stomachs which suffer through a desire to be physically appealing. We purge and don't allow our bodies the nutrition it needs. In the refresh step, we reprogram how we experience the world, our relationships, and the way we allow people to treat us and how we allow ourselves to accept.

You may have been operating in this way for a very long time. Most likely since you were 12 -15 years old when our peers, friends, intimate relationships and being popular became super important to us. There are many things that we have integrated into our social decision making. We will dive deep into what they are and how we can take back control.

1. The words you think control your feelings: Throughout this book we have discussed the importance of language. Believe it or not, it all begins the instant that we have a thought and the corresponding feeling that is created or the other way round. For example, we feel that we need to be nice to be accepted. You may immediately feel trapped or guarded with that thought. Immediately a certain frequency is emitted as you struggle to recalibrate your behavior. People will respond to you accordingly. Take a moment now to connect to that. Now try and think of

how you would prefer to behave and the frequency associated with that. I'm positive that the second one feels stronger.

2. The feelings you have control who you spend your time with.
3. The sounds, music and noises that surround you affect your heart.
4. What you watch regularly affects your feelings.
5. Your environment affects your feelings.
6. The words you speak affects your thoughts.
7. Choosing to say thank you in all situations.

There are people in our life who want to be, some who have to be and others who choose to be. Those who want to be may sometimes be beneficial like your mother or your spouse. Some may want to be but not add any value like a best friend from elementary school who has an opposing world view and takes more than she adds. While I was in London to receive my Best Podcast Host of the Year award, I met many people in real life who I've known online for a few months or years and meeting new people for the first time ever. Along with the delicious ethnic food, mastering the Tube, walking in the wrong direction for several kilometers, I began examining my interpersonal practices.

I was more conscious when I chose to say yes or no to requests for help. If I said yes, I was aware that this was a transactional choice. Not, "she'll appreciate me more if I do this" but "I am doing this and before I begin I will also ask her for something I desire". If the response to my request was no, I didn't do it.

At one point, I started to actually be grateful for opportunities to see people for who they really are, even if it meant severing the relationship. It was literally the beginning of so many more rewarding and meaningful experiences. I love speaking straight from the heart and connecting with other hearts. It's rewarding in so many ways. I received a chocolate golden award, a speaking testimonial and gained a deeper understanding of what more I must add to my vision and mission.

Application:

While I was awaiting my gate announcement at Heathrow airport, I decided to grab some lunch at Pret a Manger. There were several lines moving slowly but at one in particular, a woman was struggling with using the card reader machine. When she tapped, insert slide no matter what, the payment wouldn't register. I changed lines once or twice to get around her. Until I realized that she needed some help, help that the cashier couldn't give.

I looked over and asked, "How much is your lunch?" The cashier responded "4.48£". As I was leaving the country and needed to get the right amount of pounds, I paid for her lunch. The cashier was relieved. She was shocked and people looked at me strangely. Even if I hadn't needed to get rid of pounds I would've done the same. I wondered why she just didn't ask for help. Afterwards, she came to my table and thanked me. She started to explain that she was out of cash. I smiled and said it was a pleasure to help. Then asked if she was staying in the UK or off somewhere else. She was returning home to China and needed lunch. Interesting how thanking comes easier than asking for help.

Does this situation sound familiar? Do you not ask for help when you need it?

Be an observer in life. Do you ever wonder why you keep repeating the same patterns with different people? Did you stop wondering and just give in to what seems inevitable? What if it isn't inevitable? What if it is fully within your control? Stop and watch yourself. You watch your friends, relatives and random people on the street but have you ever stopped to watch yourself? You must be an observer and student of yourself in life. Do it objectively. Observe your thoughts and the choices to which they lead. This is the beginning of your rebirth.

I have found out so far that I do actually practice what I preach. I'm all about the pause and staying replenished in my body. It's so funny because the week I returned from London, I wasn't sure whether to expect jet lag or not. But I built it into my schedule anyway. There are even more ways to stay replenished in my body than I realized!

Ask and you will receive...It really is that simple. So make sure your question is specific and asked to the right person. Today choose your vibration. When you vibrate higher, you pull in a different crowd...in particular your inner circle. People who are humble, love hard and walk-in gratitude. When you select, know this. The highest vibrations are:

> Peace
> Love
> Gratitude

You are what you radiate. What will that be today?

Activity:

Ask for exactly what you desire and observe how it changes the way you show up.

CHAPTER 8

REBIRTH: MASTERING YOUR MINDSET

Quote: "My recipe for life is not being afraid of myself, afraid of what I think, or of my opinions". ~ **Eartha Kitt**

Main Idea: Mastering your mindset is so much more than resilience. It is the mental pivot that opens you to receiving everything you desire and pray for.

Anecdote:

Mothering is the hardest job on the planet. It hit me like an 18 wheeler in the early days after my separation being the complete emotional anchor for my children. Yes, it wasn't a sudden revelation as I had been doing that for years. Suddenly, it felt like I had to more deeply integrate my own emotional journey whilst being present with my children. Listening to how they were processing the whole situation I could literally feel their emotions in my body. The heaviness started in my heart and radiated throughout my body to the point that I wanted to be face down in a complete puddle of flowing tears. My shoulders, stomach, thighs all began to cave even though I was sitting. In the middle of the afternoon, I felt like going to sleep from their vibration. In fact, these feelings happen because each one of those emotions has a specific vibration. Dr. David Hawkins found that emotions have measurable energy. For example, peace has a frequency of 600 Hz (hertz), love has 500 Hz, fear has 100 HZ, and shame is the lowest frequency with 20 Hz. Definitely in this case, me and my child were vibing at 100 hz. I had to shift the energy. I allowed them to completely share their story and then we would do a healing session. Sometimes that meant I taught them self-massage for the affected energy centers, or we did an essentrics based exercise, prescribed a specific soak in the tub, or we ate specific healing foods. You see, I take motherhood so seriously, I study each child's vibration according to their humor. That is my default as a Tibb practitioner, intuitive healer and loving mom. I remember the day that I took my mothering to this level. Up until then, I only focused these methods on me. My rebirth began with the pregnancy and birth of my fifth child and third daughter. I needed to have a space just for me to self reflect, build, believe and trust myself again. So I began to write. I wrote about all of my research surrounding elimination communication, curing eczema, cradle cap, discovering healthy ways to cook traditional Bengali food, staying positive during arguments with your husband, how to not allow your heart to be infiltrated by constant insults from your intimate partner, how to have self-compassion, self-forgiveness, managing the mental gymnastics of helplessness and hopelessness whilst being positive for your children. All of that and so much more is what built Replenish Me ™ and Sweet Talk ™ and ultimately my coaching practice.

While our marriage definitely crumbled in the past three years, it was the beginning of the end at least seven years before that. My only choice was to be the victor. Everywhere I looked there was no help. Even the people who said that they would be there no matter what I need, had abandoned me. My parents were long gone and it was just me and Allah. I had the ultimate gift of detachment from the physical world. I had the ultimate gift to choose to vibrate higher, in peace.

Information and Application

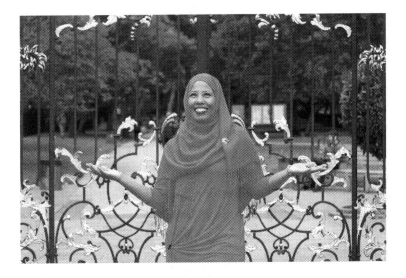

About a year ago, I was in London in October, my favorite month for retreat. While it wasn't a retreat, I was on retreat and introspective on my self-nurturing practices. I wrote a significant part of this book in the process.

This is one of my favorite pictures of all time. I decided to have a photo shoot and in the end had two! This particular day, my photographer had chosen Holland Park. When I saw the gates, I thought oh yes! Anyone who has been to London knows that this faces a very busy intersection and we literally stopped traffic. People were asking who I am. It was quite a buzz and I loved it!

You see, I struggled with wearing the color red for many years because it was a truer reflection of my personality. Truthfully before this photo the last time I had worn red was for my 21st birthday! It's the me that I hide and try to keep small. It's the voice that I allowed to be silenced and of which I actively participated in the suppression.

That day, I freed myself to just BE.

However, when I returned home, I worried and wondered whether I should or could even post any of my red goddess pictures.

- To me, it would mean having to BE the TRUEST version of me,
- it meant giving up "safety"
- it meant recognizing my Divine Feminine in all of her glory
- it meant being FREE TO BE!!!

In fact, I recoiled within so much that the very reason I was there, to receive an award, became a challenge. Let me explain...yes I physically received the Best Podcast Host of 2019, yet in my soul and the essence of my being it took having a coffee with a dear friend another 3 weeks after my return to the States!

Let's breathe into that for a moment. Are you feeling this moment of fear of showing up with me? Have you ever done something like that? You know struggle to receive recognition? Perhaps something you truly desired and totally had put your heart and soul into and then you discredit or dismiss or don't acknowledge the accolades or yourself? That's a THING for many women!

I'm here to tell you the other side of the hiding is everything you've ever desired. Lean into your WOMAN IN RED, allow yourself to be FREE TO BE, walk that talk deep in your soul.

Observe:

It's been fun observing myself continuously over the course of the years that I have been growing my business and message. Knowing the path and walking the path are incongruent sometimes. Like I know and live the concept of Sweet Talk ™ yet I find myself often shit talking to myself anyway. I discovered that my mind was a prison of energies tied to words, vibrations tied to patterns of behavior, choices resulting from both and default states refusing to relinquish power to love. I know that I don't believe in the power of the negative words that vy for attention and space in my mind. I know that love is the highest vibration after peace. I know that I have a choice in how I behave, react or not to others. I know my default states tend to lean fear rather than love. I used to fear loving myself because I felt free and detached from everything and everyone which made me feel guilty. I had been taught that loving required attachment. Does that sound familiar? So as I am writing this book my "pour into you" revolves around what goes on in my mind. I had a shocking discovery. I lacked the freedom to focus on whispering sweet nothings to myself. Do you know what I mean? With this book, I have granted myself, and invite you to join me, to have freedom to focus on pouring into myself with Sweet Talk ™. So in this book, I have walked you through the steps of Replenish Me ™: Release, Restructure, Refresh and now Rebirth.

Activity:

I'm calling you to be an observer and student of yourself. For this activity, I want you to track your menstrual cycle. Stay with me. If you are not a woman, track your emotional cycle in a month. *"I'm braver when I'm ovulating."* Was an astonishing revelation for me. For some reason, after the pause that I experience almost a complete interplanetary vacation, I take during my menstrual cycle. I return to my body in full force a week later during ovulation. That's the power required to conceive a child so wouldn't make sense to be powerful? In fact, the number one way that women give up their power is through their womb space. If we were so bold as to proclaim that, "I will not allow any man into my womb space/ vagina who does lift my vibration, honor my inner values, desire in life what I desire" the world would be a better place. There would be no fear that all women would be alone, only a guarantee that men would change drastically. I can hear the women who swear that they already do that. I'm here to tell you that you are not...not truly. Collectively humans have a fear of loneliness and even the women who temporarily stop the flow of pussy to get what they want are not doing their womb space justice or giving it its true power. Our womb space is the inner core of our personality and being. Physiologically it is protected by the groups of muscle we revere as "the core". The place where we flex our sexy abs. However, the truly sexy part is neither the exterior well toned abs nor what happens when men enter our vagina. The sexiest part is the energy with which we decide to share our soul being with another human being for cellular, spiritual and intergalactic pleasure beyond human comprehension.

During this observation period keep a journal and resist the urge to have intercourse. You can have sexual contact with only a partner who lifts your vibration, honors your inner values, and desires in life what you desire.

Here's why:

The Sacral chakra is the source of your rebirth. How much power do we give up with who we share our womb space with? The inner work is self-nurturing. In your moments alone who are you? You know those intimate moments where you boldly look into your soul. There you find yourself lingering longer each time as you lean into who you really are. Intimacy begins within. It's a spiritual thing at its core. How are you exploring who you really are? Do it through intimacy. The best part of intimacy is that the inner work surrounds self-nurturing. In its simplest form that means being a loving mother to yourself.

CHAPTER 9

REBIRTH: PHASE 2 RECEIVING AND EXPERIENCING COMPLETE JOY

Quote: "You are on the eve of a complete victory. You can't go wrong. The world is behind you." ~**Josephine Baker**

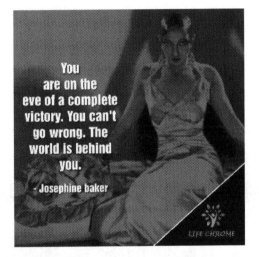

Main idea: Now that you are able to do the mental pivot, it's time to do it experiencing complete joy. Let's embody joy in your rebirth!

Anecdote:

When I was brainstorming a logo for Replenish Me ™ in 2019, I desired it to be reflective of my journey and that of my client. In fact, when I was building Replenish Me ™ I was at my lowest point emotionally, financially, spiritually and physically. It was around my birthday. I decided to go hiking with a group of women who had a hiking

Facebook group. I thought, "Perfect! I will go hiking with complete strangers. This will save me from having to reveal myself and I can just connect with nature." Each step of that nine mile trail I felt life enter back into me. The tree cover and height prevented me from using any function on my phone outside of taking pictures or videos. Complete freedom from doing and absolute being in the moment, discovery of creation and myself. Finally we reached a waterhole with a huge boulder and stopped for lunch. I set up my carrots, cucumbers, walnuts and seeds and removed my shoes. As my soles touched the rock and I looked up through the tree cover, I felt a complete rebirth as if that boulder was my personal charger. With each bite, my power surge increased. My joy was on overflow as I now stood on the rock and breathed for what seemed the first time all year. This break marked the midway point for our descent back to the parking lot. I could not wait to return home to receive my full download. Upon my arrival back home, I sat in my garage for 40 minutes writing the full 12 steps and imagining my new logo.

Those 12 steps have since distilled down to four after having coached several women in the various versions and iterations of Replenish Me ™. The logo has even evolved from the original green to a brilliant coral red maintaining the sun ray symbolizing your inner brilliance being radiated out into the world. The focal point was always on who that YOU be...the lotus flower and the reason you no longer need to be stuck. The lotus flower symbolizes rising from a dark place into beauty and rebirth, as this is exactly how a lotus flower grows directly out of muddy and murky waters and produces beautiful white and pink blossoms. It is a symbol of strength. The seed's journey is to move calmly through the darkness and into the light. Once the seed completes the journey, it blossoms into the next stage of life. That is why I chose it as my logo. I am so excited that I created it myself. The idea was born out of purity and love for what I do. Even without doing the research of the significance of the lotus flower, I felt into my soul for a visual representation of my brand. My decision to create my own logo started with a prayer and stillness. Sometimes your soul just knows, and your mind must follow without justification or judgment.

Information:

It all begins in self-nurturing. As you go through life you experience, challenges and if you allow right next to it is also the solution. The gap between the two is the self-nurturing piece. If you have not understood by now, the difference between self-care and self-nurturing is one perpetuates doing and the other being. Here is the actual definition of self-care:

The practice of taking an active role in protecting one's own well-being and happiness, in particular during periods of stress.

In health care, self-care is any necessary human regulatory function which is under individual control, deliberate and self-initiated. Some place self-care on a continuum with health care providers at the opposite end to self-care while others see a more complex relationship.

As you can see it is very reactive and includes things like: showering, brushing teeth, eating, exercising, etc.

Here is the definition of self-nurturing:

According to Dr. Jessica Michaelson, "Self-Nurture is the prerequisite to Self-Care. Self-Nurture is an everyday state of being, not a once in a while treat."... **"Nurture reflects a general attitude toward yourself, an attitude of believing you are worthy of tenderness, and able to provide it to yourself through your thoughts and actions."**

In my own words, self-nurturing is mindfully selecting the food that gives your body the optimum energy, brain performance and health. It is recognizing that your body requires sleep at a certain time and aligning your day so that you can sleep peacefully at that time. It is seeing that not only do you need to exercise but what that particular movement should do to give your body the best result that day. And when it comes to facing challenges in life, it means choosing to feel all of your emotions, even the ugly ones so that you can glean the wisdom from your emotions as well as the situation itself. When I slow down to breathe, I am able to see the obvious. Slowing down and being in the moment versus "doing" something is always the answer. Here's what I have learned:

1. Approach adversity with possibility all the way through.
2. Pause and breathe if all the answers don't surface at once.
3. Believe that there is a solution and it will all work out.
4. Look at the facts. In my case, I have received a miracle and blessing everyday since I have chosen this path.
5. I have healing to do and deserve to live an abundant life with love (spiritual love, self-love and love from a life partner)

Ultimately, I am talking about self-trust. What you don't know about me is the inner struggle and mental gymnastics it's taken me to get here! What you don't know is the daily self-doubt and hits I have endured to my self-belief. What you haven't seen is the blood, sweat and tears of my five year journey in my business and the previous 13 years to even decide to start it. What you don't know is you have to be your message to see your message. It's not all about a catching or clever mission statement and vision. Not even an eye-catching website, beautiful graphics or cool logo, it's about what we commonly known as confidence. Confidence is built not gotten.

Do you ever have things happen in life that throw you completely off kilter? Before you can even recover the next thing comes and you begin to question not only your capabilities but your capacity to endure. **It all comes down to...*You are who you believe you are. It's all about self-belief. You decide who that is and no one else.*** So firmly lean into your darkest and most difficult emotions as a matter of self-nurturing. Receive nurturing and love from yourself first and foremost. Align to your values, purpose and vision joyfully. The other side of that is also ensuring the people you reach out to for support are also aligned with your values, purpose and vision. Everyone is not on your team and discernment is so very important when you are allowing it to all happen. At this point in the book, you have *released* everything that's expected and accepted in your "culture" and have moved into clearly identifying **YOUR** values. Bearing them in mind, *restructure* your habits and choices to support them. Build and practice them daily, *refresh* your inner circle only to include the people who support them. In concert, these three steps will create the foundation for your joyful *rebirth.*

Application:

Do you believe in yourself? How do you handle your world when it spins in retrograde?

Rebirth is the freeing of the true and new self with all the layers peeled, connected only to God and the purpose for which you were created. Take off the mask you are wearing. Come out of the closet where you are hiding. Listen, from a place of compassion, to the projections of others which you have been interpreting as judgement and welcome the possibilities or goodness. Detach from others opinions. Detach from needing to be enough. Detach from fitting into a mold. Declare proudly, "Replenish Me!" Joyfully embrace the imminent lesson and value of each unpleasurable situation. Who will you rebirth as? Even more important is to know who is allowed to and deserving of walking with you in your rebirth. This is the soul level part of rebirth. In my Raise Your Vibration mini - retreat I started with the name of Allah Ar-Rahman the Merciful. Repeating words that have deep spiritual healing and meaning can protect your journey. Protection is key at this point. Protecting your heart, mind, body and soul are done through vibration, words, and actions.

Al-Wali is a beautiful Name of Allah meaning the *Protecting Friend* or the *Nearby Guardian.* All of the shades of the Name are sourced in the concept of closeness. Wali is the opposite of an enemy, which I thought was an interesting way to qualify it. But it makes perfect sense. The definition of enemy: *a person who feels hatred for, fosters harmful designs against, or engages in antagonistic activities against another; an adversary or opponent.* An enemy is not disengaged. An enemy is very engaged. So the opposite of that is to be engaged as well. A Wali is not neutral. Someone who stays neutral when you need their support is closer to your enemy than your friend. So it's not the neutral folk, it's the people we call ride or die. The people who got your back, and your sides, and your front. The people who will go to war for you. That's the receiving part. The other side is experiencing joyfully.

How do you experience adversity joyfully? Change your words! Get curious about what lessons it has to offer you.

Activity:

1. Make a list of your ride of die people who deserve to be with you in your rebirth. Identify and qualify what makes them eligible.
2. How do you experience joy and where do you feel it in your body? Let's repeat the Feel Into Your Body Activity from Chapter One.

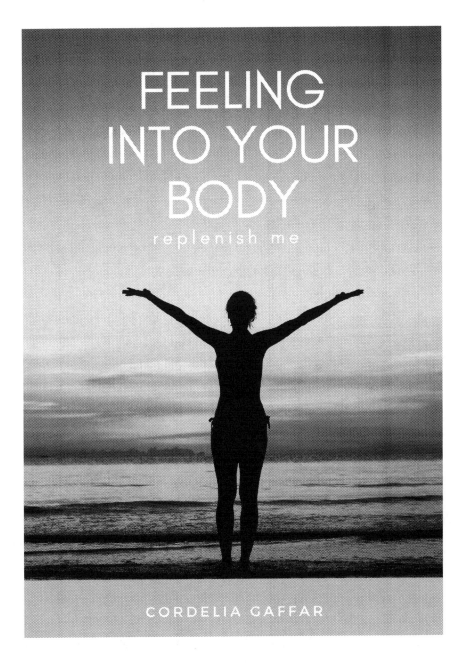

FEELING IT INTO YOUR BODY

self expression

receiving love, compassion

willpower, passion

emotional and financial support

sexual energy and belief to do anything

NEGATIVE EMOTIONS IN YOUR BODY

despair, grief

other people's burdens

fear, anger

repression, abandonment

shame and guilt

frustration

CORDELIA GAFFAR | ©2020

NEGATIVE EMOTIONS
≈
DOWNWARD EMOTIONAL FLOW

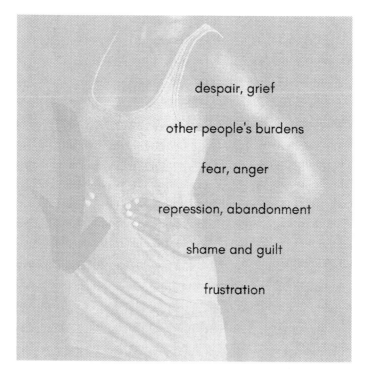

despair, grief

other people's burdens

fear, anger

repression, abandonment

shame and guilt

frustration

WHAT'S THE STORY YOU HAVE BEEN CARRYING?

In the space below, capture your guilt, shame, judgement or any other
story you have been carrying since your childhood.

_____

_____

_____

_____

_____

_____

_____

_____

_____

_____

_____

_____

_____

_____

_____

_____

_____

_____

_____

_____

_____

REFLECTION

Reflect on how your story has played out for you so far.
Describe below how you have been showing up and whether it's true.
Then describe how you can change or rewrite it.

_____

_____
_____
_____
_____
_____
_____
_____
_____
_____
_____
_____
_____
_____
_____
_____
_____
_____
_____
_____
_____

CREATING YOUR MAP-BRAIN DUMP

Using what you have written so far, perform a brain-dump below, on your top three desires to turn your life around.

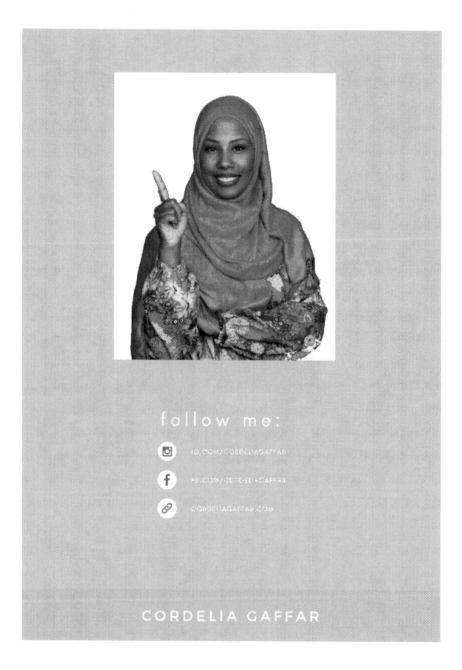

CHAPTER 10

SHOWING UP POWERFULLY

Quote:

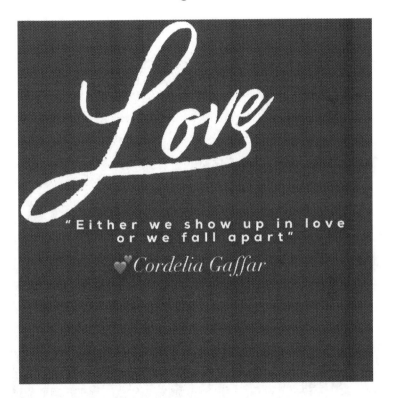

Main Idea:

Showing up powerfully is all about love from the inside out. This is a quote from a talk I did on Allyship, a topic I knew nothing about, blending my transformational Replenish Me ™ process with the hard topics of race, diversity and inclusion, and invited people to be students of themselves.

Anecdote:

I had to call myself out in the middle of my Raise Your Vibration Mini Retreat. During the two hour session we learned about vibration and how to change it on a cellular and spiritual level. When we got to the part about voice, I shared an old story that I had forgotten was there which is still operating on a subconscious level and caused a change in my physical state. I had to stop and walk myself through a lesson being witnessed by this intimate group of 7 women. The objective was to seek for MY TRUTH and create a new reality with my words by reprogramming my muscle memory. That means create a new choice.

As you grow up there are different experiences which become defining moments. Although we often hear that most of them happen before the age of seven, the truth is that the ones that shut down your voice and define your adulthood happen between the ages of 10-15. This is the age of reinforcing your life path. Do you remember an incident which you in the moment consciously decided, "I will never ever tell anyone my true heart's desire" or "I will never show myself true self again", or maybe "Now that I know no one cares or sees me, I will do whatever it takes to be someone else"? There are many variations of what we choose in that moment. In my case, I choose to silence my voice and redirect my energy towards what other's find more acceptable attributes of my personality and being. Yesterday I was confronted with showing up powerfully with my voice and overcoming it IN THE MOMENT or to continue to hide! Wow! Can you imagine my absolute FEAR to be in that space again after decades of hiding AND in front of my clients at my own event? I did it! I did it for me, for the healing of my voice, for the reprogramming of my muscle memory and by extension for the women now witnessing and holding space for me. It was the most powerful redefining I have ever experienced and one of the women said, "that is great leadership and a powerful model of what to do when we experience that, Thank you!"

It was the most powerful part of the whole retreat!

I learned that you can take a moment and pause for the cause of reprogramming no matter what is happening. The most important thing to remember is that you always have an opportunity to heal. You always have a choice to reveal yourself or to remain hidden. Choose what gives you life and helps you to lean deeply into growing as a leader. So my question to you today is are you seeking your truth? ...Truly desire to show up powerfully? Sometimes showing up powerfully is being vulnerable in front of the very people you are leading. Be the example of what diving into your deepest emotions looks like. You may get it conceptually but there is nothing like having a real time palpable demonstration complete with blood sweat and tears. I sang a capella in public for the first time in over 30 years. I literally freed my voice. As Sade says, "I am a soldier of love".

Information within an Anecdote

It feels so freeing to just move my hips in so many different ways to music that makes my heart happy and my mind laugh. I am free with every other woman around me...so many women wining up and exploring the limits of their hips without any sexual intention. This is how it feels every time I have a Replenish Me ™ workshop. No ogling men's eyes. No judgemental women's eyes. Only women leaning into their bodies freely to experience emotional freedom and healing. None of us as victims of violence, war trauma or any "severe" emotional situations that may come to mind. No, we are women living our lives and using our voice in a world that normalizes varying levels of emotional abuse of women enforced by company, local, national and global policies which edify the immature male ego whilst demonizing the woman's basic right to walk down the street. As I look back on my journey, I always dance to feel that freedom and healing. My journey of showing up powerfully is an intricate awakening emerging into corporate America whilst completing the coveted College Degree. Being a very spiritual being struggling with my human experience literally colored by being a Black woman. Here are some examples of what my work environment was like at 23.

"I'm a partner here, you cheeky b*tch!"

Or

"You can look the other way so that we can push this through, right sweetheart?" with a wink.

These are some of the colorful comments I recall when I used to go head to head with partners in the law firm where I worked as the billing coordinator at the beginning of my financial career, to when I served as controller for a small IT start up. Always being patronized and belittled for enforcing company and federal regulations!

A woman's path to showing up powerfully is about her voice. It is about the choice to give in to the status quo or to be true to herself. Women are described as celestial beings. For example, Venus is both a goddess and the name of a planet. We have idealized Mother Theresa and Florence Nightingale, both caregivers and pious women. These are all beautiful examples of "purity". In real life, that looks like us playing the good girl, i.e. not talking back or speaking up. On the more earthly and sinister end, we have been described as Sirens in mythology, seducing men to their deaths. Delilah, Jezebel and concubines were all sexualized, which is a complete misunderstanding of the power and purpose of femininity and sexual energy. Back to my story, that is being patronized being called "sweetheart" and not taken seriously as a professional enforcing the financial and legal parameters. At the core, it is the woman's voice that's been silenced...my voice was silenced so many times. There are times when I felt hopeless and froze. Toxic shaming can be overwhelming on many levels. It sounds like this in my head, "I am invisible, my words don't hold the same weight as a man or white woman, why did they even hire me?, I hate my life, I am going to numb from all this pain!" Can you relate? What do you hear in your head? Each human being should be respectful towards the other no matter the way she speaks, looks or dresses. Women dress for themselves not for others because ***news flash*** we don't objectify ourselves. As I look around the room that day in the Dominican Republic, I welcome the fact that my sexuality is the companion of my spiritual self and self-discovery. Leaning into the power of my existence by allowing myself to feel deeply into my body, especially my womb space in communion with other women, I feel free to be. From my studies, I know that women trap negative emotions in the thighs, lower back, stomach and are represented in breast, ovarian and cervical cancer. On the chemical level, it wears on our adrenal glands which run the show metabolically and send us signs in minor bulges, weight gain, insomnia, or oversleeping. We have been taught to be detached from our bodies so the correlation between insomnia for a week, excessive sugar tendencies and gaining 15 pounds, sudden belly bulge becomes a thing to fix. The conversation in our head is '*OMG I'm fat!*' not '***What's been going on for me lately? How can I stay ahead of it and get my systems back in balance***'. We've been sold that we need to fear our bodies and have "them" constantly monitor our most intimate parts. What if you could turn it around just by trusting your body and being a student of it and nurturing it the way we are taught to others? Imagine taking pleasure, sanctuary and joy in your own love manifest as your body? Feel into this as a blank canvas ready for your creative expression. It is a blend of taking back ownership of your sexual story, body, heart, mind, and sexuality/spirituality as a whole going forward. Yes, spirituality! What happens when we have sex? Usually a child is created without all of the modern precautions. Their souls come from the spiritual realm and yes we even pray for children. I will dive more into that later.

So how is sex spiritual? I was familiar with the commercialized kamasutra but not the true meaning of it or that there are several traditions that have a similar teaching. In July 2001, I chose to become Muslim as the result of a 5 year spiritual journey after my parents had died in consecutive years. Yes, I found it intriguing. I learned about the rest of the prophets, Jesus, Mary may the peace and blessings of Allah be upon them all. However, I really desired to know more about what it means to be a Muslim woman. I not only found out that Islam came as a liberation for women in a society where the infant girls were buried, women were considered chattel and having daughters were a disgrace but there's more! Yes, Islam gave women rights to land, wealth, education,... and wait for it.....rights over their own bodies down to full books written about intimacy in marriage. The responsibility of marrying a woman was to protect her lineage, heritage and SEXUALITY. That's the true reason I became Muslim! A way of life that protects and gives voice to your spiritual core as a woman. In the Quran, it is said that the 1% of mercy Allah left on Earth was placed in the woman's womb. Even with the veil of shame lifted through my new chosen life, I still had an internal struggle between my sexuality and my outer appropriate behavior. The Muslim women I met had women's only dance parties but excessive music and dancing are considered shameful. That means that only during wedding season or the two Eids did we meet up. That was a shock to my system as I always used both to decompress from my day. How did I survive? My *Ill Na Na* or self-expression whispered through my writing. Sexual energy is our creativity. My words are birthed and my voice shows up powerfully, soulfully pulling through the gifts from the spiritual realm meant for this world.

Without showing up powerfully, it is quite simply emptiness, the epitome of a closed off part and silenced voice. For myself, I did all of the appropriate things and ticked all of the boxes by my choosing to marry. I wasn't being frigid but modest, right? Besides as a Black woman, for me marriage was sexual freedom not bondage because no one would question whether I knew the father of my children. *That actually happens!* In fact Islamically having sex every four days is recommended because it solidifies the love and compassion in a marriage. However, in most marriages it is weaponized by the wife or the husband and becomes a thing withheld. Besides sex has one purpose, to procreate, right? Have you ever wondered why marriages dissolve and the connection disintegrates? The connection between the physical self and the emotional self is in our loins. All throughout Islamic tradition, the divine is bridged in this world through emotions. When a man and a woman consummate marriage, there is a prayer said to presence God in their intention of combining their bodies in the physical form to welcome the blessing of perhaps a child through intercourse.

Here I will introduce the opposite of my journey. What happens when a Black woman shows up with balanced feminine and masculine energy rather than just the accepted docile feminine. Foxy Brown, the first Black female rapper of Trinidian parents from Brooklyn, New York. She was dubbed *Ill Na Na, which means awesome vagina in patois,* by Nas a male rapper from Queens. Their paths were very different while her career suffered and she was bounced between producers, who were all men, scraped for contracts and to produce albums. Meanwhile he is considered the grandfather of rap and just produced his 13th album successfully after a 30 year career. I'm mentioning her to demonstrate what the single Black women's career, sexuality and path to discovery looks like. Juxtapose to me, a good girl mindful of my reputation and measuring my voice, it appears she suffered more. Yet even though most of my life I hid my truer self and she boldly owned her Divine Feminine, my suffering has been silent and the same as hers. She has been in and out of jail with "anger management issues", suspended licenses and at the age of 41 like at the beginning of her career is featured on one of the songs on Nas' new album. I started my business at the age of 43 and have been in and out of emotional bondage. When this sexual power is consistently crushed, it is the voice of the woman being silenced, also known as repression. The repression becomes anger and eventually rage. Anger is the most demonized emotion yet the biggest gift to humanity. It awakens a wisdom within our core that can make the world a better place. I used my anger and rage to continue my business even after two and half years of disappointment, being unsupported at every turn and even being threatened with loss of security and love. At the end of the day, I had to take a stand for my values. During my year long period of cognitive dissonance, it leaked out in emotional splatter. It took me to Bali where I could speak freely on stage. When I returned, I went flat overwhelmed with self-doubt and judgement. In Foxy Brown's story, her rage pushed her into compliance. My rage ran me into the mountains last year to deal with the fact my ***Divine Black Feminine, my term for my truest self-expression,*** is not well received. As you see the opposite of my story yields the same ending.

What I know is that moving my hips freely with women wining up is my sexual identity, a power so strong that the world feels off kilter when she speaks. The world may say that it represents something to objectify. The truth is she is the Divine Feminine. As I step more and more into my power and truly begin to show up more powerfully and bold, I question my choice to lessen my expressiveness around my body and sexuality. I fully recognize and accept that I can. Lean into your rage and other dark emotions, allow yourself to walk that talk deep in your soul. Release your voice. Pause and truly allow yourself to feel them for the full 90 seconds they are present. Then speak from the depth of your soul...be Free to BE! Start your path to showing up powerfully.

Application:

So let's break down what is happening with our hips, sacral and root chakras here. At 23, I was not aware of nor did I have the regular conscious release practices that I do now. However, I did go out and dance with my friends regularly or in my apartment as I got ready for work. I can say that even back then dancing was more for my mentally release and physical decompression than for being social or dancing with another person. What I know now is that being in your body is a very important part of the body, mind and soul connection and daily healing. As we revisited in the previous chapter, the activity on Feeling Into Your body, there is a lot going on from our diaphragm to our hips. In particular in this chapter, I want to focus on our hips and genitalia. This is so very important to healing and almost never integrated into personal development.

Although we think of a woman's genitalia as only the vagina, there is a whole world of parts we are missing. Anatomically that section is called a vulva. This includes: mons pubis, labia, clitoris, urethral opening, and vaginal opening. In 2017, a study done by Hebernick D et al stated that only 18% of women reach orgasm with vaginal penetration alone - the rest require clitoral and vulva stimulation! Are you a woman who has never reached orgasm? I invite you to explore your vulva. Above and beyond the vulva, I would include the solar plexus, lungs and breathing in general as part of a woman's full sensual experience and sexual pleasure. The activity I'm introducing below could be viewed as controversial yet I ask you to welcome the possibility that it may be your healing. This can be used as a daily self-nurturing routine and especially when practiced with loving intention. Ground yourself into your body with dance and sensual exploration, prayer, spiritual reading and then being very selective with your nutrition to start your day. For the nutritional piece, I recommend calcium magnesium and super B complex after breakfast and lunch. Having practiced this for several months, my periods came in seamlessly, no skin changes i.e. pimples, no severe mood swings and no bloating.

Tips and Activity

Sensual grounding activity.

If self-pleasure is new to you, start with your clothes on and eyes closed. Explore your body slowly and use your breath to slow you down. Whilst inhaling, place your hands on your face. Exhale whilst caressing your cheeks. As you work your way down your body, neck, décolleté (the area between the neck and breast), breast, shoulders, arms, elbows, fingers, diaphragm, stomach above your navel, navel, immediately below navel, vulva, thighs, buttocks, thighs, knees, knee caps, shins, calves, ankles, instep, heals and toes. To lessen friction and make it more pleasurable you may use extra virgin olive oil, coconut oil, almond oil (optional to enhance pleasure use a drop of your favorite essential oil). If you do not have any of these things the first time do not allow it to be a barrier for you. Do it anyway!

Caress and touch yourself slowly and freely. The first time you may use a timer for 5 minutes and increase the time by 5 minutes until you reach a full 30 minutes. The objective is to explore, acknowledge, experience the touch of your own skin for personal pleasure. Touch as many parts slowly and deliberately as possible in the time allotted. By the time you reach 30 minutes, you will know which areas you enjoy exploring and ways to manipulate for optimum pleasure. Once you are comfortable, make written notes of what feels best. Become a student of your sensuality and reclaim your body, pleasure and sexuality.

You're welcome!

So now what? You will know once you repeat this activity daily, although not recommended during your menstrual cycle as that is a sacred time of cleansing. You will find that this activity will rewire your brain and muscle memory of your soul self. In my case, I started the week that I spoke on Allyship and that was the best talk I had ever given in my life. I got rave reviews and connected with more people than ever before and afterwards. It was a gift that kept giving. My business turned around dramatically, opportunities sought me, my entire world of everything I ever desired flooded me.

Detaching powerfully from what is expected and accepted of you in every way with every fiber and cell of your body is the direction transforming your heart so that you can transform your mind. Truly and deeply loving yourself is the best part!

ABOUT THE AUTHOR

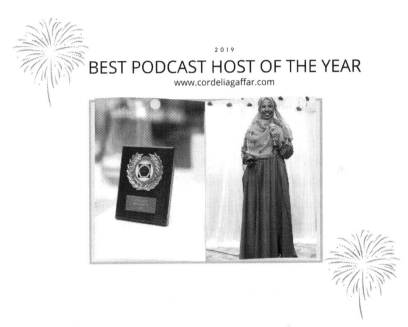

2019
BEST PODCAST HOST OF THE YEAR
www.cordeliagaffar.com

Cordelia Gaffar is the Emotions Opener Transformation Strategist guiding leaders to use their darkest and most difficult emotions to show up powerfully.

In 2020, Cordelia Gaffar was nominated for Top National Influencer by the Success Women's Conference, Sexy Brilliant Ambassador and inducted into the Global Library of Female Authors by Ona Miller and hit best seller again with the **1 Habit for Success SmartFem Edition**. **Detached Love: Transforming Your Heart So You Can Transform Your Mind** is her seventh book and fourth solo book. Cordelia is the Best Podcast Host of 2019, for her Free to Be podcast, and the ACHI magazine Volunteer of the Year and finalist for Top Influencer and Orator of the Year. She is best-selling co-author of **America's Leading Ladies: who positively impact the world** with Oprah Winfrey and several dynamic women.

Once upon a time 25 years ago, whilst watching her parent's health decline and the increase in their prescriptions, she threw herself into studying and applying herbal and plant medicine to her life so that she would not be at the mercy of the health system. She made her life's work to know her body so well that she could detect any imbalance immediately. 18 years ago she was able to immediately detect imbalance after the birth of her second child. She was able to release the weight of her mind, body and soul. All those years of study and implementing practices for herself is what she has poured into Replenish Me ™.

After leaving her corporate career as a controller for an IT start-up, she homeschooled her six children which involved coordinating activities in the homeschooling community, running girl scout and boy scout troops and much more. She emerged as an author sharing how to self-nurture in **The Guide How to Get Started with Workout Around My Day.** She began coaching women in her community, deepened her craft with continuing research and study in nutrition, fitness, spiritual practices and overall emotional wellness. Most recently she has been selected Ambassador of Peace by INSPAD and Director for the USA chapter and other collaborations.

Currently she is studying to be certified as a Tibb Practitioner. She is the Founder of Replenish Me ™and the official sponsor of She Phoenix, Femme Phoenix Ltd in South Africa. Even with all of her accolades her biggest brag is being a homeschooling mom of six children. *As seen on America Meditating Radio, on South African radio 786, The Sexy Brilliant Show, Fox News and British Muslim TV.*

Connect with her on social media and on her website.
https://www.cordeliagaffar.com/
https://www.linkedin.com/in/cordelia-gaffar/
https://www.facebook.com/groups/ReplenishMeGroup/
https://www.youtube.com/c/CordeliaGaffarWOAMD
www.instagram.com/cordeliagaffar
https://www.facebook.com/ReplenishMeRetreats
https://www.facebook.com/FreetoBeShowandPodcast

Printed in the United States
by Baker & Taylor Publisher Services